Social Skills for Nursing Practice

Social Skills for Nursing Practice

Second edition

Peter French

PhD BA DipN STD RGN RN RMN CPsychol
Department of Nursing
The Chinese University of Hong Kong
Hong Kong, China

CHAPMAN & HALL
London · Glasgow · New York · Tokyo · Melbourne · Madras

Published by Chapman & Hall, 2–6 Boundary Row, London SE1 8HN, UK

Chapman & Hall, 2–6 Boundary Row, London SE1 8HN, UK

Blackie Academic & Professional, Wester Cleddens Road, Bishopbriggs, Glasgow G64 2NK, UK

Chapman & Hall Inc., One Penn Plaza, 41st Floor, New York NY10019, USA

Chapman & Hall Japan, Thomson Publishing Japan, Hirakawacho Nemoto Building, 6F, 1–7–11 Hirakawa-cho, Chiyoda-ku, Tokyo 102, Japan

Chapman & Hall Australia, Thomas Nelson Australia, 102 Dodds Street, South Melbourne, Victoria 3205, Australia

Chapman & Hall India, R. Seshadri, 32 Second Main Road, CIT East, Madras 600 035, India

Distributed in the USA and Canada by Singular Publishing Group Inc., 4284 41st Street, San Diego, California 92105

First edition 1983 by Croom Helm Ltd

Reprinted 1985
Reprinted and published 1989 by Chapman & Hall
Second edition 1994

© 1983, 1994 Peter French

Typeset in 10/12 Palatino by Columns
Printed in Great Britain by St Edmundsbury Press, Bury St Edmunds.

ISBN 0 412 47840 4   1 56593 228 5 (USA)

A catalogue record for this book is available from the British Library

Library of Congress Cataloguing-in-Publication data available

Contents

Contents

Contents

Preface

All interpersonal processes may have constructive or deteriorative consequences.

Carkhuff, 1969

The motto for the second edition remains the quotation taken from Carkhuff because it is still true that all members of helping professions should be encouraged to consider what attempts they make to ensure that their social interaction is constructive rather than destructive in its effect. Nursing has a heavy responsibility in this context because it is carried out from the standpoint of a relatively long-standing, intimate, social relationship. It will be constantly reaffirmed in this text that the feature most characteristic of nursing is the shared interpersonal experience of the nurse and the patient. Yet it is still evident from research findings that the acquisition of skills for interpersonal relating has been woefully neglected in nursing curriculum during recent years (Melia, 1981; Macleod Clark, 1983; Birchenall, 1983; Faulkner, 1985; Wattley and Muller, 1987; French, 1989). It is not the case that nurses do not acquire social skills during their preregistration preparation but rather that the process of acquisition occurs haphazardly and principally in the context of socialization in clinical practice.

In this scenario the interpersonal processes can have deteriorative consequences for the nursing student, and may well be the cause of much of the stress of learning in the practice setting (Birch, 1978; Parkes, 1980a; 1980b). It has long been argued that under stress nurses will learn to protect themselves from conflict and inadequacies by adopting methods that can be detrimental to the patient's progress (Menzies, 1960).

This book has been produced in the firm belief that all people have the potential to improve their skills for interpersonal relating and that nurses, because of the nature of their work, have a responsibility to acquire and facilitate the acquisition of social skills to improve the quality of nursing care. It is also the contention in this book that social skills may be taught and learned like any other skill. Crute *et al.* (1989) have recently demonstrated improvement in interpersonal skills using particular microteaching methods with health visitor students. The similarity between psychomotor skill and social skill may be closer than many would at first appreciate. Argyle (1969; 1972) lists several characteristics that are shared by both motor and social skills:

1. They are directed towards some end; they have an intended outcome or aim.
2. There is selective perception of cues. The performer looks for specific information in the environment that is associated with the skill.
3. There are central 'translation' processes. The information received is converted into appropriate action. As this becomes more efficient the process becomes automatic.
4. The existence of motor responses. Social skills are also portrayed by body movements.
5. There is feedback and corrective action. As each action is carried out this provides additional information, which allows modification of action to increase efficiency.
6. The timing of responses is important for efficiency. The sequence and production of responses must be carefully managed so that they are co-ordinated and appropriate.

Bearing these comparisons in mind it is not too difficult to see that social skills can be acquired in much the same way as psychomotor nursing skills. Indeed there are several critical features of social skills learning that have been recommended.

The simplest is that the person who wishes to perform a social skill efficiently needs to know: (i) indicators that suggest that the skill should be deployed; (ii) how the skill is to be carried out; and (iii) when the skill should be discontinued.

Dealing more specifically with interpersonal skills Crute *et al.* (1989) recommend a microteaching method of skill acquisition, which consists of four stages:

1. Skill analysis, understanding the strategies and component parts of the skill and the theoretical rationales for adopting them.
2. Skill discrimination, evaluating the effectiveness or ineffectiveness of the skill.
3. Skill practice, practice in adopting the skills.
4. Focused feedback, evaluation of performance based on self assessment and independent feedback.

The first of these stages of skill acquisition is important in the context of this book. A common issue in the development of social skill is the appropriateness of theory or technical-rational knowledge to the development of skills that many nurses argue are most amenable to experiential learning. There are several reasons why it is not idiosyncratic to contribute to the development of experiential learning by using a textbook as a medium for facilitation. They are all related to the process of reflection in the experiential learning cycle:

1. Reflection can be promoted by the existence in the person of a cognitive conceptual framework.
2. This framework also provides a language that enables the communication of experience of interpersonal transactions.
3. The discussions in this book can provoke the development of individual perspectives.
4. Many of the reflective activities suggested in this book encourage the participant to observe and test out the ideas presented in this book in real life.

The information in this book is presented as an adjunct to experiential learning programmes and structured exercises in interpersonal relating. Egan (1990) seems to support this approach when he says that a plan of learning for interpersonal relating should include 'Working knowledge', which is the 'translation of theory and research into the kinds of applied understandings that enable helpers to work with clients', and 'Skill', which he describes as the 'actual ability to deliver the services'.

This book will be of little use if it does not incite the reader to engage in some sort of active participation in simulated and real-life interpersonal transactions and then to reflect on the quality of these transactions and the potential for personal development. If this occurs then the reader as a consequence may be more prepared to help others to develop their own interpersonal skills in the context of nursing practice.

There are, however, some words of warning that should be heeded as the reader peruses and considers the contents of this book.

The first is that social skills can become very contrived and mechanistic if they are adopted as a set of procedures and techniques. While there are guidelines in this book that recommend steps or stages in social skills, the primary goal for the reader is to acquire personal strategies that incorporate the recommendations in this book where they are found to be helpful and effective. The performance of the skill is not an end in itself, it is the needs of the patient and the nurse which should be paramount, as well as the need for both parties to be human and humane.

A second issue is related to the simulated practice of social skills. Often we practice social skills in a contrived and relatively safe situation that only models some of the features of real-life situations. It is important, however, that the reader tries to use these skills in nursing practice, knowing that there is always scope for improvement in interpersonal transactions.

A final point is related to the initial difficulty in acquiring skills. Social skills, like all other skills, can be awkward and unwieldy at first. Rehearsal, constant use and reflective thought will refine these skills so that they can become a usual part of the nurses' practice repertoire. Just as we can give an intramuscular injection, drive a motor car or swim without thinking through every action in the sequence, social skills can also become automatic. Some nurses argue that carrying out some social skills is too time consuming. There is, however, the argument that the use of these skills decreases the workload by facilitating nursing practice and preventing the problems caused by persistent unmet social and emotional needs (Bridge and Macleod Clark, 1981). Suicide, attention-seeking, non-compliance, learned helplessness, aggression, anxiety and hopelessness, are some examples of time-consuming problems that can occur as a result of neglect of social and emotional needs.

This book attempts to begin the process of social skills learning in several ways. The first is concerned with identifying those nursing activities that can be called social skills. This text can be viewed as a catalogue of nursing social skills. The second aim is to introduce a body of knowledge associated with the practice of social skills. The text will refer to other work on the particular topic, sometimes without discussing it in further detail. The work is presented in the hope of providing a key to a wider body of knowledge. Students of nursing social skills are strongly advised to read the texts that are commonly cited, so that they can acquire a full appreciation of the issue under consideration. This book is presented in the hope that it will provide an impetus for reflective practice and the development of social skills in the nursing curriculum.

Acknowledgements

I would like to acknowledge the following people for their various contributions to this book: Phil Neely, Medical Photographer, Darlington Memorial Hospital and Maria Wong Sau-Bing, photographer, The Chinese University of Hong Kong; Jennifer Hunt and Diane Marks-Maran for permission to reproduce the history sheet shown in their book; Jean Roch for the publication of the interview schedule that she designed; The Chest, Heart and Stroke Association for the reproduction of their Word and Picture Chart. Mr J. Guttridge and Mr R. B. Combes formerly of Bethlam Royal and Maudsley Hospitals for permission to reproduce sections from the *Guidelines for the Nursing Management of Violence*; Career Track International and Scandinavian Training School for the use of some of their ideas; and Tim Hardwick and Rosemary Morris for their invaluable and tactful advice, guidance and patience.

CHAPTER 1

Introduction to a transactional view of nursing

LEARNING OBJECTIVES

You should concentrate on being able to:

1. Give a definition of nursing in your own words that will summarize the work of the nurse in any situation and which emphasizes the transactional approach.
2. List the stages of the scientific method.
3. List variations of the theme of the scientific method.
4. Describe each of the stages of the process of nursing.
5. Discuss the process of nursing by applying it to a minor illness that you have dealt with at home.
6. Describe briefly why the process of nursing may take on varying forms in different nursing specialities.

THE BASIS OF NURSING

Nursing is the activity of assisting a human being, who depends on fellow human beings to maintain a state of health and overcome health problems or deviations, in the context of a continuous interpersonal transaction.

This may be achieved by a professional or a natural approach. The professional approach requires a great deal of knowledge and skill because of expectations and demands placed by society on the nurse practitioner who occupies this position. The natural situation involves an untrained person who uses skills gained during ordinary life experience (and who may have vested emotional interest in the dependent individual) to achieve nursing aims. Examples of the latter include mothering, altruism, and caring for ill relatives or friends.

Several points should be borne in mind when interpreting the definition set out above. To some extent all human beings are dependent on each other to meet their needs. The major concern here is with those individuals who require assistance with the meeting of needs that they normally carry out for themselves. Henderson conveys this sentiment when she says:

> The unique function of the nurse is to assist individuals, sick or well, in the performance of those activities contributing to health or its recovery (or to peaceful death) that they would perform unaided had they the necessary strength, will or knowledge. And to do this in such a way as to help them gain independence as rapidly as possible.

Henderson,1966

The second point that should be emphasized here is that nursing is seen to be an interpersonal transaction – something occurring between two people. The word 'transaction' has been chosen because it is: 'Relating to negotiating, conducting, performing, or carrying on, as an act or process; pertaining to an interplay' (see 'transactional' in Campbell, 1989).

Both nurse and patient participate in the nursing process, the actions, thoughts and feelings of one influencing the actions, thoughts and feelings of the other. Nursing is not carried out **on** patients but **with** them (Figure 1.1). It is even reasonable to suggest that the awareness of the patient's equal involvement should be borne in mind whether the person be unconscious, or demented, or uncommunicat-

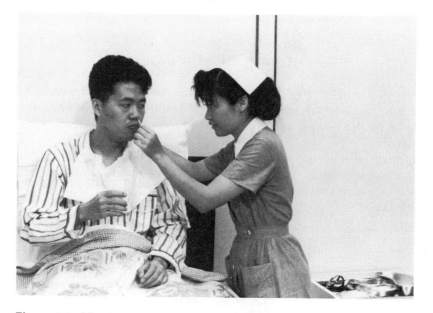

Figure 1.1   Nursing is carried out not **on** a patient but **with** him.

ing, very young or elderly, or delirious, or asleep, or mentally disordered or severely neurologically impaired. If this is not clearly retained, patients are in danger of losing their distinctive human qualities and the nurse may see them as just objects. Frequently this transactional quality of the relationship can be used in itself as a therapeutic measure. Burton makes the following relevant comment:

> The relationship that develops will vary in intensity and the length of time required to establish it will vary too. However, it is essential that there should be a relationship, an interaction or feeling between two people, before real help can be given.
> *Burton, 1965*

A final point to be made about nursing is that one of the people in the relationship is dependent and the other relatively independent. The patient is rarely dependent of his own choosing and this situation is potentially one of unequal power distribution. It is too easy for the independent person, the nurse, knowingly or unknowingly to take advantage of this. This dependent/independent situation, however, sets the scene for the characteristic nature of nursing. It is also important to notice that the aim of the nurse in most cases is to bring the individual to a state of relative independence and thus make his or her existence unnecessary with respect to that individual. Few occupations can involve themselves in personal relationships with such potential intensity on a continuous basis, yet the nurse/patient relationship must always end if the nursing care is to be successful.

NURSING IN A SYSTEMATIC AND ORGANIZED WAY

How then can the nurse carry out this activity in a systematic and efficient manner? Nursing has been called a science and the scientific approach to life has become a dominant feature in our society. The scientific method aims to add to our knowledge of the world by using the following tried and tested sequence of events:

1. Identifying the problem to be investigated.
2. Collecting relevant information.
3. Proposing a solution to the problem.
4. Testing the solution.
5. Abstracting general principles.
6. Applying to new situation and identifying new problems.

This is the hypothetico-deductive model. This form of disciplined approach is predisposed to several manifestations: (i) the research method; (ii) the project method and problem-solving approaches, e.g. problem-orientated medical records; (iii) the nursing process; and (iv) goal-oriented care. It may be useful here to look at the research method as a variation on the theme that is of current relevance to the nursing profession. This involves:

1. Defining the problem.
2. Studying the literature.
3. Planning the method of investigation.
4. Testing the proposed method (pilot study).
5. Collecting the data (information).
6. Analysing the data (interpret the data).
7. Drawing conclusions from data.
8. Recording, reporting and communicating to others.

Compare this with the scientific method; how do they differ? The problem-solving approach has led to the nursing process in which the nurse must: (i) identify a specific problem; (ii) record accurately all details and observations that pertain to the stated problem; (iii) outline clearly a plan of approach to solve the problem; (iv) indicate when the problem is resolved or if it remains unsolved (Ulisse, 1978). Accepting that the patient's needs and difficulties are problems, the nursing process can now be described. This process not only provides a description of the work of the nurse, but also provides a framework and a system of terminology in which the activity of nursing can be discussed overtly. A five-stage process of nursing has been identified (Taylor *et al.*, 1989; Stanton *et al.*, 1990), which consists of the following steps: (i) collecting information about the patient; (ii) assessing the patient's needs; (iii) planning care; (iv) implementation; and (v) evaluation.

Collecting information about patients and their situations

This involves obtaining as much information as possible about the person as an individual and the needs, difficulties and problems that they may have. The nurse should attempt to be aware of their habits, preferences, physiological functioning, social relationships, feelings and thoughts and past in so far as patients or others are willing and able to impart this information. Furthermore, the patients' signs and symptoms complement this picture in that people, when classified as patients, have some actual or potential disturbance of health state, which brings them into contact with the nurse.

Assessing the patient's needs, difficulties and problems

Some authors combine the previous stage with this one. They are separated here in the hope that this stage will be seen as a decision-making activity rather than a mere collecting process. Here, on the basis of the relevant information collected systematically, two decisions are made. The first decision is to identify what the problems and the patient's requirements are. The second decision is to identify which requirements are more urgent or more important than others: here the needs, difficulties and problems are placed in a hierarchy of importance. In adopting the interpersonal approach to nursing, it is necessary for the nurse and the patient to make these decisions together wherever possible.

Planning care

Now that the patient's needs and difficulties have been identified, the nurse should draw up a plan of action. This involves stating the needs and difficulties and aims or goals with respect to these needs. In other words, the nurse should ask what state in the patient do the nurse and patient want to achieve realistically. These goals set the criterion or measure that will help determine how far these needs have been met or the patient has been helped with the difficulties. The resources that are available to help the patient, such as equipment, manpower and environment, should be assessed. Finally, the nurse can state what she will **do.** The nurse here commits herself to some action to help remedy each difficulty or meet each need.

Implementation

This involves carrying out activities and procedures, co-ordinating them with the plans of other professionals, gaining the assistance and co-operation of the patient and communicating all this information to others. This book will be concerned particularly with interpersonal aspects of these nursing actions.

Evaluation

Here the nurse sees how far the patient has been helped by her activities by comparing the state of the patient with the goals set in the plan. Inherent in this is an assessment of how effective and efficient is the nurse's performance. As a result of evaluation, some needs and difficulties may disappear or emerge or the hierarchy of importance may change. This process may be carried out either subjectively or objectively and by one person or a team of people. In the latter case, the whole process must be carried out by a team of nurses and, in order to maintain communication between team members, this should be carried out in an objective form.

The patient as the focal point should be re-emphasized, lest his or her role is allowed to become insignificant. The patient should be seen as a team member in all situations. One of the major problems in team and institutionalized approaches to nursing is that the identity of the person, the individual that this whole system is geared to, is in danger of being ignored.

The above process remains the same whichever speciality the nurse works in. The only difference is that the people who are the subject of the application of the process can differ markedly. They may be very young or elderly, they may suffer from physical disorder or mental disorder, they may have disorders specific to men or women. Whatever the situation, it is the predominant needs, problems or difficulties that change, not the nursing process.

REFLECTIVE ACTIVITIES

1. Try to remember if the definition of nursing given here applies to nurses you have met as a patient or observer.
2. Ask a patient what nurses do for him or her that he or she particularly appreciates.
3. Next time you have a problem to solve see if you can apply a scientific method or problem-solving approach to find a solution or course of action. Does it work? How is this different to the way you might otherwise have solved the problem?
4. When you carry out nursing duties try to keep a single day's detailed record of the activities you were engaged in. How does this compare with the nursing process model?
5. When somebody at home or work becomes ill, e.g. with influenza, see if you can apply a simple version of the nursing process to help him or her. What feelings or problems does he have? What can you do about them? How do you decide when he or she does not need your help anymore?
6. If you are involved in a nursing speciality and are currently experiencing this area (e.g. psychiatry or community nursing), see if a local training school will let you see a film on the role of the nurse in a surgical or medical ward. How does your list of activities differ from those on the film? Are there any activities that do not fit into the nursing process model? Do you consider them nursing activities? How do you decide what are nursing activities?

SELF-EVALUATION TASKS

1. In your own words write down a definition of nursing without looking back at the text.

2. List the stages of the nursing process.
3. Write a few lines on assessing patients' needs and difficulties. Refer to the text to check your answers.

CHAPTER 2

Assessing the person's needs and problems

LEARNING OBJECTIVES

The nurse should be able to:

1. Define the term human functioning in terms of man as a 'biopsychosocial' being.
2. List three sources of variation in human functioning.
3. Give examples that illustrate each of the sources of variation in human functioning.
4. Define the terms: needs; problems; actual problems; potential problems.
5. Draw up a hierarchy of human needs as described by Maslow (1954).
6. Briefly describe the relevance of Maslow's hierarchy of needs to needs' assessment in nursing practice.
7. Draw a diagram to show the complex inter-relationship between needs, problems, areas of human functioning and variations in human functioning.
8. Understand the value of conceptual nursing models for the process of nursing assessment.
9. Define the phrase 'nursing observation' so that it describes the aim and underlying processes characteristic of this activity.
10. Describe a model of perception with reference to sensors, transmission channels, area of appreciation and sensory filter.
11. Define the terms 'bottom-up' and 'top-down' processing.
12. Define the word 'attention'.
13. List eight factors that influence attention.
14. List five activities that contribute towards observational skill.

THE NEED FOR ASSESSMENT

The basis of nursing in an interpersonal framework is the full acknowledgement of the existence of, and mutual co-operation between, two human beings – the nurse and the patient. In order to appreciate the context in which nursing takes place, it is important to understand how these two basic units of the interpersonal process function. One constant feature of socially skilled action is the continuing assessment of the effect one is having on the other person. To become proficient in this assessment as a professional practitioner it is necessary to understand how human beings function and how changes in functioning may be observed. A further requirement of any skilled action is knowing **when** to carry out the skill. This often means identifying a change of state in another human being that indicates that the social skill is appropriate. In addition the skilled practitioner needs to identify when the skilled action is no longer required and this also requires an assessment of the state of the other person.

Two approaches will be adopted in this analysis of human functioning. The first looks at human beings as if they all functioned in a similar way, compartmentalizing human functioning in global terms. The second approach accepts the fact that human functioning varies from one person to another and in one individual from one moment to the next.

HUMAN FUNCTIONING

Man is a complex collection of cells organized as a whole and carrying out those activities that characterize living things. These activities (adapted from McNaught and Callander, 1971) are:

1. Irritability: the ability to respond to changes in the environment.
2. Contractility: the ability to move.
3. Nutrition: the ability to secure materials from the environment and incorporate them into own body structure.
4. Metabolism: the ability to undertake complex constructive and destructive chemical processes.
5. Growth: the ability to replace or add to existing structures.
6. Respiration: the ability to take in and use oxygen and remove and excrete carbon dioxide.
7. Excretion: the ability to remove waste products from the body.
8. Reproduction: the ability to produce replica organisms from the original organism.

As living organisms humans are in a state of constant exchange with the world that exists beyond the boundaries of his body. Many of the activities that characterize living objects support this assertion. This clear-cut distinction between humans and their environment is, however, not as simple as it sounds. Humans are composed totally of elements coming from their environment (i.e. they are a product of their environment). All of the materials that make up the human body return at some time or other to become part of the environment again (through excretion, elimination or death).

Humans also build their own environment (parts of their environment are a product of their activity). The room, this book and the place we live in, are all human-made. An interesting point to ponder is that every other human being is a constituent of each human being's environment. Piaget's analysis of man's interaction with his environment is particularly attractive. Piaget (1952) points to the fact that every event that occurs between humans and their environment is, at one and the same time, an action of humans upon their environment and an action of the environment on humans. Humans and their environment are in dynamic equilibrium with each other. They share their existence; they do not exist in isolation from each other. Each human is a biological being and, since other humans are a part of his or her environment, he or she may also be considered a social being.

An analysis of this type has been suggested by Roy (Riehl and Roy, 1974), who sees humans as 'biopsychosocial' beings. To understand human functioning fully their experience can be categorized into three broad areas: (i) the biological (physical or physiological); (ii) the psychological; and (iii) the social. The biological area is concerned with the structural, physical and chemical phenomena occurring within the boundaries of the body. Study of anatomy and physiology deals with this aspect of human functioning. The psychological area is concerned with human mental activity, private experience and their effects on human behaviour. Social functioning focuses on a human's involvement with others, the life that is shared with other human beings. In order to understand human functioning fully it is necessary to study biological, psychological and social aspects of life in equal proportions. However, it should always be remembered that these categories are formulated to assist our understanding of the human being. Humans function as whole entities, not in separate parts.

One can also see that when changes occur in one area of human functioning they are likely to bring about changes in the other areas because of the simple fact that humans function as a whole. Thus problems in one area can bring about problems in other areas. Take the example of what is commonly thought of as a biological problem, influenza. The body has been invaded by virulent micro-organisms. The lining of the nose and throat becomes inflamed, the individual coughs and sneezes to remove the irritation. The body directs its defensive resources to the removal of the micro-organisms. The person is, however, encouraged to hold his hand over the mouth or cover the coughs and sneezes with a handkerchief so as not to trouble other people (social effect). As the person becomes more fatigued he or she cannot be bothered with other people and may even become isolated from others as he or she takes to bed. This person now depends on others to supply food, drink, medication and to perform activities such as turning out the light, making the bed and opening the windows. The person will often moan or cough loudly to attract the attention of others so that they may sympathize with his predicament.

At another level being ill costs money, involving buying special medicines or losing time at work. We also change roles for the time that we are ill, e.g. someone who is known as the librarian becomes 'the patient'. In addition to these social changes several psychological changes occur. Emotional changes may be observed; we feel unwell. With influenza, depression is a common phenomenon. Discomfort and pain may be experienced or the person may become frustrated or worried. The person may find it difficult to concentrate or may not find the energy to become interested in any physical or mental pursuits (motivational change). At the height of a fever the patient may suffer hallucinations or illusions (perceptual changes), suffer confusion or become delirious, all of which indicate changes in psychological functioning. It is safe to assume that in all 'illnesses' all areas of human functioning are in some way affected.

HUMAN VARIATION

Up until this point it has been implied that all human beings function in a similar fashion and to some extent this is true. The common elements of human functioning provide much of the raw material for the scientific study of biology, psychology and sociology. While having many things in common, human beings are each unique. What adds complexity to the study of human functioning is the almost infinite number of ways in which each human being differs from any other human being at any one moment in time. Each person looks different, thinks differently, has different abilities and associates with his or her fellow human in different ways.

Even when one considers human anatomy, which is often thought of as invariant, we find that there are differences in body size and shape, veins, arteries and nerves may differ in their exact position in relationship to neighbouring structures, people may have extra structures (e.g. an extra kidney), or have organs or parts of the body missing. One person's appendix may be the length of a little finger, while another's may be as long as a knitting needle.

In the study of psychology, differences between individuals are encapsulated in the concepts of personality, intelligence and creativity in particular. Many of the topics of sociology, such as role, class, status and culture, point to differences in individual social behaviour that can characterize a human being, making him or her distinct from another. Biological variation compels the descriptive anatomist to deal in average measurements, the surgeon to be prepared for the unexpected, the clinical radiologist to remain open-minded and the impresario to be on the look out for unusual individuals who might prove to be commercial assets. There is not the space here to describe in any depth the disciplines of anatomy, physiology, psychology or sociology. There are many books available that more than adequately cover these subjects; some are suggested in the list of references at the end of this book.

A second and important source of variation is that associated with time. Individuals differ in themselves from year to year, from day to day, even from minute to minute. Emotions are an obvious example of differences in ourselves that we may all be aware of. Some days we may feel bright, others slow and sluggish. At one moment we may be miserable and the next moment, after receiving good news, we can suddenly become elated. We change from day to day just because we add to our stock of experience. The study of human development looks at human change that occurs throughout the lifespan. In Piaget's (1952) terms one can also detect differences in human thinking that occur on the basis of each interaction with the environment. Each perception of the outside world allows us to assimilate information that involves its incorporation into our already existing set of thoughts. Each moment that a person lives he or she is altered by the environment. Body structure and functioning also change because of a human's dynamic interaction with his or her environment. Body composition changes from day to day as chemicals from the outside world are incorporated into its structure and others are rejected (i.e. digestion and excretion respectively). Even physiological efficiency may alter from day to day and, as we become older, parts of our bodies degenerate and become less able to complete the functions ascribed to them.

A third source of variation in human behaviour concerns environmental change. Because of humankind's close relationship with the environment one would expect that as the environment changes, so does he or she. The degree of alteration in functioning is usually commensurate with the degree of difference between the new and the old environment. The amount of previous experience with the new environment will also influence the alteration in functioning brought about by the change. One example of substantial environmental change is hospital admission. The person with no previous experience of hospital life may undergo several functional disturbances: becoming anxious; finding it difficult to sleep; feeling lost; not knowing how to react to others; making mistakes; feeling insecure; not eating or stopping going to the toilet. The reader may wish to consider how his or her behaviour and body functioning may change if he or she were at this point in time suddenly transported to some primitive African village. Hospital admission is in many ways a similar experience. Some changes in environment are not too difficult to adapt to. This may be exemplified by the patient who must visit hospital regularly or has been an in-patient on several previous occasions. The patient is less likely to experience severe functional changes as the environment becomes more familiar.

NEEDS

A need can be described as a lack of some necessary factor or condition that maintains adequate biological, psychological or social functioning. A need can be seen as some deficiency interfering with normal functioning. These deficiencies compel the person to action that aims to nullify the effects of the lack.

James (1975) describes two major groups of needs, balancing needs and progressive needs. Balancing needs are those that maintain a state of equilibrium, either too much or too little of the relevant item causing rectifying action. An example is the need for water: a lack causes behaviour that aims to secure water, while too much causes body homeostatic mechanisms to release water from the body. The second type of need, the progressive need, is that in which the goal continually moves on as it is satisfied at each level. One example could be the need to be productive or creative. As one thing is created the person may yearn to produce something better or more complex. As needs become stronger there is a tendency for the individual to become increasingly more concerned with the restoration of stability. The person pays much more attention to stimuli relevant to the activity of procuring the requirement. There is also a tendency to ignore those stimuli that are not associated with this aim. When a need becomes really strong the individual becomes so single-minded in his attempts to satisfy the need that it becomes something of an obsession. This increased focusing of energy and strength of rectifying action as the deficiency becomes more severe has been called drive (Hull, 1943).

It is worth differentiating between 'needs' and 'wants'. The distinction lies in the fact that needs **must** be satisfied while wants can be put off without any serious disruption of human functioning. It is clear, however, that in humans there are examples of requirements that are difficult to categorize as needs or wants. Where an individual requires a house in terms of shelter this is probably a need. A caravan and a mansion are both forms of shelter but could one say that the mansion is required only to meet needs for shelter? Humans have become so complex in their requirements that it is difficult to tell if motor cars, televisions, the telephone and even toilets are needs because in some cases their removal disturbs human functioning.

Since man can be viewed as a biopsychosocial being, needs may be categorized into social, psychological and biological needs. There is a general tendency in nursing theory and practice to emphasize biological needs and pay comparatively less attention to psychological and social needs. Indeed the distinction between psychological and social needs is not made, and the widespread use of the term 'psychosocial' indicates a reluctance to understand fully these aspects of human functioning. Often the term 'psychosocial' betrays the fact that the user cannot make the distinction between these two areas of functioning, yet the clear categorization of biological aspects from all others is invariably made. It is worth making a distinction between aspects of individual mental functioning and behaviour, and those concerning human relationships, particularly when assessing and meeting human needs during nursing activities. Table 2.1 provides an outline of several human needs under these categories to give the reader some idea of their variety. The needs given in the table are by no means always clearly distinct from each other and the list is not exhaustive. It may be apparent that many needs are closely related and cut across categories (e.g. relief of sexual urge and sexual intercourse). One must remember, however, that these are artificial aids to understanding and, as stated earlier, humans function as whole beings. It is easy to see therefore that some needs will obviously be closely related. It should also be remembered that there is often variation in the terminology used to describe a single need. An

Table 2.1   Needs Checklist

Physiological	*Psychological*	*Social*
Food and Water	Freedom from unpleasant feelings	Security with others
Oxygen	Acquire pleasant feelings	Acceptance by others
	Sensory variation	Recognition
	Curiosity	Affiliation
Freedom from injury	Self respect	Parental needs
	Acceptable self-image	Sexual intercourse
Elimination of waste	Self-actualization	Love (give and receive)
Stable temperature	Order	Communicate with others
Relief of sexual urges	Harmony	Space, territorial needs
	Beauty	Competition
	Formulation and preservation of beliefs	Access to shared resources
	To learn	

example is the need for sensory stimulation, which may also be described as freedom from boredom, the need for novelty or sensory variation.

Hierarchy of Needs

The concept of a hierarchy of needs, proposed by Maslow (1954), is helpful in highlighting some of the important principles of needs assessment in nursing practice. Maslow suggested that motives, and by inference needs, are ordered into levels of importance according to the priority that they command (Figure 2.1). It is proposed that motives lowest in the hierarchy will be precipitated first and must be satisfied or they will remain dominant. When needs low in the hierarchy are satisfied, needs at the next highest level will appear and demand satisfaction. If one examines the hierarchy of needs it can be seen that, according to Maslow's conception, in general, biological needs must be met first, social needs next and psychological needs last.

An important feature of Maslow's theory is that two useful guidelines for nursing practice may be extracted. The first relies on the principle that needs lowest in the hierarchy should be met first. This provides a tool for needs assessment. Once needs are identified they can be placed in order of importance with respect to the amount of nursing attention required. We can thus confidently place a need for oxygen as a more important consideration than sensory stimulation (occupational therapy). It is obvious that if a person cannot breathe he

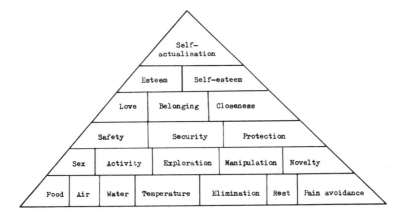

Figure 2.1 Maslow's hierarchy of needs.

or she will have little time or inclination to be involved in other pursuits and may also find it difficult to eat, wash and sleep. Even though this may be painfully obvious to the reader, without this sort of assessment nurses often make mistakes in trying to meet needs that are inappropriate or which are trivial at that point in time.

The second principle for nursing derives from the point that once needs are met, new needs will emerge. Some needs may not even appear until needs lower in the hierarchy are met. The pattern and priority of needs is thus constantly changing. The nurse must constantly reassess the patient's needs and their position in the list of priorities. If this is not carried out, nurses will find themselves assisting patients with needs they no longer have. An example is the careless nurse who carries on feeding the patient who can manage alone, ignoring pain or depression in the same person, sometimes with disastrous consequences. Constant evaluation or reassessment is thus a very crucial stage of the nursing process.

Problems

At this point it is important to remember that all human beings have needs and it is possible to think of human functioning as a process in which we spend our lives meeting needs. In addition two seemingly contradictory points concerning the meeting of human needs are important. The first is that, to some extent, all human beings rely on each other to meet most of their needs. The second is that, in general, people are able to initiate action to meet their own needs. Bearing these two points in mind, it is possible to say that nurses are required when people cannot meet their own needs independently. The help required is usually above and beyond the amount of help normally required by another to meet needs. It is at this point that we begin to call people 'patients' and their needs 'problems'. It is easy to see that the person in this situation becomes dependent on the nurse if effective life-functioning is to be maintained. This applies equally well to preventative care as well as to curative approaches or long-term support and care. It also becomes equally applicable whatever the specialist area, hospital or community, whether it be older or younger age groups. Bower described admirably the relationship between a need and a problem:

> A problem is an interruption in the individual's ability to meet a need, it is a difficulty or perplexity that requires a solution. . .when family is not able to meet basic needs, requires assistance or does not recognize unmet needs, a problem exists.
>
> *Bower, 1977*

If nursing is to be seen as an interpersonal phenomenon one should never forget that the other major partner in the relationship, the nurse, will also be influenced by his or her own needs and problems. Nurses should be able to recognize and assess their own needs, to avoid them interfering with providing help for the patient. The nurse's needs can easily conflict with those of the patient. Take, for instance, the nurse's need to help other people. This may conflict with the patient's need to become independent of help, if the nurse persists in doing things for the patient who no longer needs help. Nurses are meeting many needs in carrying out their work, some of which are inconsistent with helping patients. The instrumental aim of gaining money in employment is in itself unrelated to any true spirit of altruism. Nurses must then become aware of their own needs and ensure that they do not interfere with the patients' progress.

In Figure 2.2 are shown the major areas of assessment of human functioning and how permutations of the three dimensions described above give examples of the complex decisions that must be made

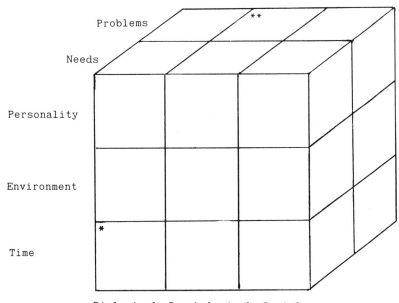

Figure 2.2 The variety and complexity of human assessments.

when assessing other people to enable nursing care to be given. The figure shows that nurses can identify needs and problems in three areas of human functioning, taking into account variations due to constitutional and personality factors, time and the environment that patients finds themselves in. One can take for example the area marked on the diagram with a single asterisk. This area in a three-dimensional sense points to the fact that there are biological needs that are alleviated or made worse through the passage of time. An example could include the fact that all people experience hunger that varies at different times of the day depending on when the previous meal has been taken. The box marked with two asterisks represents a situation in which the person is experiencing a psychological problem that is influenced by personality factors. An example of this would be the patient who becomes severely anxious, finding it difficult to alleviate his or her own anxiety, the problem being added to by the fact that he or she is generally a 'nervous' person anyway.

MODELS FOR NURSING ASSESSMENT

Nurses throughout history have come to shape and communicate to others the nature of the job that they do. In essence, they have accumulated a knowledge that is passed on to the next generation. The knowledge and understanding that nurses have developed is represented in each nurse's mind by several concepts. A concept can best be described as a collection of beliefs about a particular aspect of the world. The concept in the context of this discussion is 'nursing'. The idea of concept is based on the psychological theory that the person creates a representational model of the world in the mind, which allows him or her to reflect on the world and not just respond to it.

We obtain our personal conceptual models by learning. This learning may be acquired in a formal way by education, or informally by our observations in our daily lives. Models represent a way of acquiring concepts from people who have tried to construct formally a representation of the real world. For example, like a house on a model railway set or a popular board game, or the architectural plans for a house, they try to emulate the real world by representing some critical features, in a scaled down form, so that they may be manipulated for the purposes at hand. All of these examples represent a house without actually being one. Models for nursing practice try to do the same thing, they try to simplify something that is too complex to be handled in one go by one human mind. The difference, however, is that conceptual models try to construct representations in our minds rather than provide tangible replicas of the concept. So a nursing model helps us to think about nursing by trying to present a framework of knowledge that originates from the thinking (conceptual formulations) of other nurses.

Nevertheless, like the examples of the model houses given above, conceptual models for nursing should not be taken to be exact replicas of the world of nursing. However, their is evidence that each individual nurse will construct his or her own working concepts based on these models. Indeed one psychologist argues that each human being is a natural scientist, who takes in information (data) and checks it against his or her beliefs about the world (Kelly, 1955). In this way the person develops his or her own constructs or models of the world. This suggests that in order to formally share our knowledge we need scientific models but that we each individually adopt the relevant aspects into our own constructs. Nursing is a complicated process and nursing models help us to think about it. Much of the discussion that follows represents a selection of conceptual models, some nursing some not, which can help nurses to arrive at their own constructs about the assessment of patients.

IDENTIFICATION OF PROBLEMS

This part of the chapter will present four models of nursing to demonstrate alternative theoretical perspectives that can be adopted to organize the decisions that the nurse will make when identifying the patient's problems. The first to be described here is the Activities for Living Model (Roper *et al.*, 1990), which helps us to understand the components of normal life that can be disrupted in our patients. Gordon's (1987) Functional Health patterns provides a similar view based on the patients 'lifestyle', while the Systems Model (Neuman, 1982) encourages us to consider stressors as a major factor in patient assessment, and a Conceptual Framework for Nursing (King, 1981) reminds us that the personal, interpersonal and macrosocial aspects of a patient's life must be taken into account.

These are at least 20 models that have been documented and the following represent just four examples to give some idea of the contribution they can make to the identification of the patient's problems (e.g. George, 1990).

ACTIVITIES FOR LIVING MODEL

The person's needs and problems can be analysed in terms of activities for living (Roper *et al.*, 1990). The elements of this model derive from a 'model of living'. They comprise a set of everyday activities that healthy persons carry out relatively unaided. It is considered that deviations from health interfere with the person's ability to carry out these activities unassisted. By definition, it is because the person needs assistance with these activities that the person has a serious health problem and also can benefit from the skills of a professional helper or nurse. The activities of living are outlined in Table 2.2 and this provides a useful checklist of the areas that can be considered when collecting information about a patient's needs and problems.

One of the interesting tenets of this model is that the patient is undergoing change associated with a particular stage of his or her lifespan. This should be taken into consideration when assessing the person. In addition the model emphasizes that each person's activities of living may be evaluated on a continuum from dependence to usual independence. At different times in our lifespan our 'normal' dependence changes. For instance, normal dependence is different when we are infants, to when we are adult and when elderly.

GORDON'S FUNCTIONAL HEALTH PATTERNS FRAMEWORK

This model relates to the previous model in that it proposes a set of health-related behaviours that are representative of the persons lifestyle, as a guiding framework for nursing assessment. Some of them are similar to the activities for living and some are not. A comparison may enable the reader to come to a conclusion about the

Table 2.2   Activities for Daily Living

---

1.   Keep the body clean and well groomed and protect the integument.
2.   Select suitable clothing, dress and undress.
3.   Eat and drink adequately.
4.   Rest and sleep.
5.   Move and maintain desirable posture (walking, lying, sitting and changing from one to the other).
6.   Eliminate by all avenues of elimination.
7.   Breathe normally.
8.   Maintain body temperature within normal range by adjusting clothing and modifying the environment.
9.   Avoid dangers in the environment and avoid injuring others.
10.   Communicate with others in expressing emotions, needs, fears or feelings.
11.   Worship according to one's faith.
12.   Work at something that provides a sense of accomplishment.
13.   Play or participate in various forms of recreation.
14.   Learn, discover, or satisfy the curiosity that leads to 'normal' development in health.

---

best presentation of these mutual concerns of the patient and the nurse. Nurses collect subjective and objective data, using assessment skills, to determine the person's health status on the basis of 11 functional health patterns. The skills that nurses use include observation, questioning, interview and counselling techniques. The functional health patterns described by Gordon (1987) can be described in the following way:

1. The client's health and well-being and how health is managed.
2. Food and fluid consumption relative to metabolic need and indicators of local nutrient supply.
3. Excretory function (through bowel, bladder and skin).
4. Exercise, activity, leisure and recreation.
5. Sleep, rest and relaxation.
6. Sensory-perceptual and cognitive patterns.
7. Self-perception pattern and perceptions of self (e.g. body comfort, body image, feeling state).
8. Role engagement and relationships.
9. Client's satisfaction and dissatisfaction with sexuality and reproductive capacity.
10. General coping pattern and effectiveness in stress tolerance.
11. Values, beliefs (including spiritual), or goals that guide choices or decisions.

Perhaps it is noticeable that Gordon's model includes more psychological and social perspectives on lifestyle. We are encouraged to ask more questions about the person's thoughts, values, beliefs, satisfactions and dissatisfactions, self-concept, roles, relationships, stressors and coping behaviours.

This is an important orientation in the context of social skills because it is a strong contention that many of these issues can be sensitive areas for the patient; they require some self-disclosure and the best way to arrive at a true understanding of these issues (notice I do not use the words data collection!) is by the use of counselling skill.

NEUMAN'S SYSTEMS MODEL

This model views the patient or client as a behavioural system, a developing individual and an interactive process at one and the same time. The model emphasizes holism – that the human being must be considered as an integrated system not a set of parts. This model emphasizes that the whole system of the 'human person' is disrupted by stressors that act to destabilize this human system.

The nurse's aim is to assist the patient towards optimum 'wellness' by helping the person to prevent or cope with these stressors. In order to do this they must identify these stressors with the collaboration of the patient.

Neuman encourages us to consider four key concepts in this model. They are humankind, the environment, health and nursing. Humankind is a system of interrelated functions, physiological, psychological, sociocultural, developmental and spiritual. Environment may be described as all those influences on humankind that may be positive or negative in their outcome as stressors. Health is conceptualized as a continuum from health to illness. Nursing is seen to be a positive influence in a human's environment that is concerned with the achievement of optimum wellness.

This model is useful because it reminds the nurse that assessment should take account of the patients' human functioning, the negative effects of the environment in which they normally live (for health promotion) or the environment in which they are currently living (for care planning), the health status of each person and the positive or negative contributions that the nursing can make to the person's health status.

Neuman also reminds the nurse that our main aim of nursing assessment is to come to conclusions about a person and his or her environment as a whole. In this way we may avoid dehumanizing the patient by being more concerned with the patient's liver, mind, walking, milestones, or blood gases than his or her humanity. It is also useful to consider that Neuman's model should also be applied to families, small and large groups as well as individuals.

KING'S OPEN SYSTEMS FRAMEWORK FOR NURSING

This model is like the previous model in that it describes nursing in a systems framework (Figure 2.3). It also asserts that the focus of nursing is the care of human beings. This model is very helpful, particularly in the context of social skills because the three systems that provide the major framework for the model, are based on the person's social transactions (King, 1981). The three systems are: (i) personal systems; (ii) interpersonal systems; and (iii) social systems.

A study of social skills for nursing practice pays particular emphasis on the personal and interpersonal systems. The personal system is similar to the concept of man in Neuman's model. It encapsulates concepts of perception, self, growth and development, body image, time and space. It is concerned with the person as an individual. Concerns with the person as a social interactor provide for King's interpersonal systems. Here the major concerns are persons functioning with another person (a dyad) in a threesome (a triad) in a small group or a large group. The important issues are interaction,

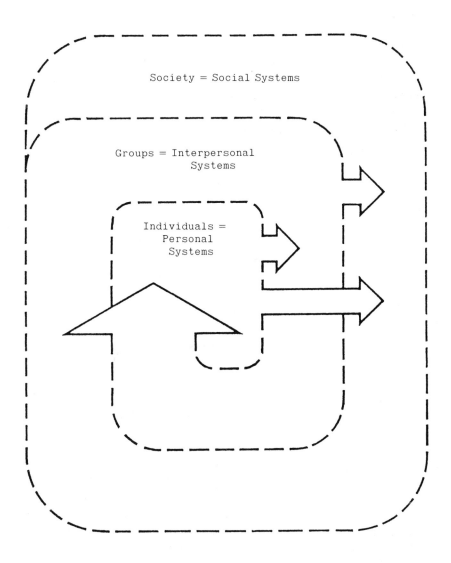

Figure 2.3   King's open systems (1981).

communication, transaction, role and stress. These concepts are more fully developed later in this book. The social systems are related to macrosociological issues. Imogene King also proposes a theory of goal attainment. Her eight axioms about goals in nursing are particularly relevant to the following discussion on patient assessment. They are (King, 1981):

1. If perceptual accuracy is present in nurse–client interactions, transactions will occur.
2. If nurse and client make transactions, goals will be attained.
3. If goals are attained, satisfactions will occur.
4. If goals are attained, effective nursing care will occur.
5. If transactions are made in nurse–client interactions, growth and development will be enhanced.
6. If role expectations and role performance as perceived by nurse and client are congruent, transactions will occur.
7. If role conflict is experienced by nurse or client or both, stress in nurse–client interactions will occur.
8. If nurses with special knowledge and skills communicate appropriate information to clients, mutual goal setting and goal attainment will occur.

These axioms can also be taken to describe the 'climate' in which nursing assessment should take place. The purpose of assessment is to identify problem areas and feasible outcomes or goals. King helps us to remember that the assessment of patients is undertaken in partnership with the patient and with the aim of establishing shared goals.

ASSESSMENT STRATEGIES

Models of nursing

The models of nursing indicate areas in which the patient's problems and needs may be described. It is crucial that for each patient the problems are stated from the patient's personal perspective. If nurses complete sentence starters such as, 'Mr Hardisty's problem is that he. . .', or 'Sally Smith needs to be able to. . .', they can ensure that they are remaining patient-centred. Research has indicated that nursing practice may not always be patient-centred (Mitchell, 1981; Swinder *et al.*, 1985; Hurst, 1985; Robertson, 1987; French, 1989; Reed, 1989). A simple approach like this to identify problems and needs may help avoid this situation. Mayers (1972) suggests that problems may be of two types, actual and potential. Actual problems are those present at the time of assessment. Potential problems are those that have a high risk of occurring if no preventative action is taken, e.g. pressure sores, wound infection. Actual problems often take priority and the patient is likely to be the person who understands them best. Potential problems may seem less significant but are equally important because of the often disastrous long-term effects. The assessment of long-term problems depends more on the knowledge and experience of the nurse and it is generally the nurse who suggests them.

Patient profiles

A common method of assessing patient problems is to use a detailed
checklist to produce a patient profile. There are several forms of
interview schedule, which can be used to construct individual patient
profiles. Some are described in the section on interviews in this book.
There are many in the literature on the nursing process and an
example is given in Table 2.3 from Mackie (1979) to give some flavour
of the type of problem assessment method that may be used. When

Table 2.3   Patient Profile (Phase 1)

1. Sleep
(a)   Usual bedtime:
(b)   Hours of sleep per night:
(c)   Do you need to get up during the night?:
(d)   How many pillows do you require?:
(e)   If unable to sleep, what do you do?:
(f)   Do you have a nap during the day?:

2. Hygiene
(a)   What bathing facilities can you make use of?(i.e. the bath, a shower, etc.)
(b)   Do you have dentures?: (Top/bottom/partial)
(c)   How do you care for your teeth/dentures?:
(d)   What are your usual bowel habits?:
(e)   Do you have any bowel irregularities?:
(f)   What are your usual bladder habits?:

3. Eating
(a)   Were you on a special diet at home?:
(b)   How much do you normally drink in a day?:
(c)   Types of fluid you prefer:
(d)   Any fluid dislikes?:

4. Ambulation
(a)   Do you normally have any difficulty walking?:
(b)   Do you use any walking stick? (Give examples):
(c)   Do you wear glasses?:
(d)   Do you use a hearing aid?:
(e)   Do you smoke? (How many per day?):

Social/Interpersonal Data
  1.   Do your relatives or next of kin know you are in hospital?:
  2.   Do you mind discussing your hospitalisation with them?:
  3.   How often do you see your family?:
  4.   How far away do they live?:
  5.   Do you expect them to visit you?:
  6.   Does anyone have a key to your home?:
  7.   If alone, are you worried about pets, cancelling orders, water pipes,
        paying the rent, etc.?:
  8.   Do you do your own shopping and housework?:
  9.   When did you last see your GP?:
 10.   What tablets were you taking at home?:

Source: Mackie, 1979.

using these profiles it is as important to remember a few important points. The first is that patient profiles are only a guide to the major problems that the patient needs help with since they may not always consider every actual or possible problem the patient may have. A second point to remember is that collecting information in this way can become an automatic routine. Nurses should not allow history-taking and the patient-profile interview to become so significant that they prevent them from making realistic decisions about the patients' problems. A third point to bear in mind is that some profiles are restrictive and are often biased in the areas of patient functioning that they explore.

One should always assess a profile to see if it covers all three areas of human functioning. The nurse should also use her experience to see if the information collected misses a common patient problem. This should be reported to the authority responsible for the production of the patient profile so that it can be modified. If problems are identified in the patient but are not covered in the profile, the nurse should find a place on the profile to include such findings rather than omitting them because they are irrelevant to the particular questions asked on the interview schedule. A further point, which is perhaps the most important, is that profiles and interview schedules are useful tools but are not always essential to the process of assessment. Schedules counter ignorance and human fallibility, but where the nurse has a good working knowledge of needs and problems she should feel free to adapt and amend any elements of an interview schedule or proformer to investigate and include the individual needs and problems of the patient. The last point about interview schedules and profiles is that they become a dangerous distraction if they become too elaborate. Information collection can become complicated and a lengthy form-filling exercise can interfere with the provision of care. However, the less elaborate a profile or schedule becomes the more necessary is the knowledge and skill of the nurse to ensure an accurate assessment. Thus paperwork can be reduced if nurses develop greater skill and knowledge with respect to the estimation of needs and problems of other people. In the context of this book, it is particularly important to identify the patient's needs for communication, so that the social skills that may be used to meet these needs can be employed. Ashworth (in Bridge and Macleod Clark, 1981) demonstrates how this may be achieved by describing the planning for communication with patients in the intensive care unit.

Observation

An additional method of collecting information in order to assess patients' problems is observation. Observation in nursing should be considered as the intentional use of the processes of perception to collect information about the patient. Observation can collect information about biological, psychological and social functioning and this commonly involves the observation of human behaviour. Indeed if one adopts the idea that behaviour is 'any observable activity in the organism' as do behaviourist psychologists (Watson, 1925), then most nursing observation concerns itself with human behaviour. One exception is observation of the patient's environment. Observation can also be thought of as a social skill on two counts. The first is that most nursing observations are carried out in close physical proximity to the patient being observed and, in some cases, direct physical contact occurs. As such, there is a possibility that the nurse's behaviour will influence the patient's behaviour. We do not normally tell the patient that we are counting his or her respirations for this very reason. The patient's pulse rate can also increase if the patient is attracted to the nurse or if he or she is exceptionally frightened of her. Even this simple act of touching can increase the pulse rate just because a stranger is engaged in this intimate activity. Some observations actually depend on social interaction between the nurse and patient. Conversation, questioning and interviewing all give information that cannot be elicited by passive or non-interactive observation such as visual observation on its own.

The second way in which observational skill can be seen as a social skill is by viewing it as an essential component for the efficient performance of any social skill (see Wilson-Barnett, in Bridge and Macleod Clark, 1981). When carrying out social skills one must constantly collect information about changes occurring in the other person. Rapport and feedback are both concepts that depend on an ability to collect information and interpret aspects of the other person's behaviour. Nurses must also become more aware of themselves as well as the effects they have on others. Self-awareness is essential to skilled social interaction. In order to understand the processes involved in observational skill it is useful to explore theories of perception and attention.

A MODEL OF PERCEPTION

A very simple model or representation of the perceptual process consists of a sensor, a transmission channel and an area of appreciation or decoding centre (Figure 2.4). The sensor, which represents one of the human sense organs, is sensitive to particular energy variations that have the capability of carrying information. Our sense organs include the eye, the ear, the olfactory bulbs in the roof of the nasal cavity, the taste buds in the tongue and the touch,

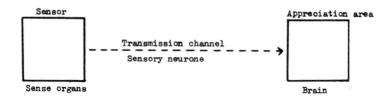

Figure 2.4   A model of perception.

temperature and pain receptors in the skin. Each of these human sensors has specialized neurones that are excited by the presence of a particular energy form. The energy forms that our sense organs are susceptible to do not represent all the energy forms available in our environment, and each sense organ only responds to one or two types of energy at most. The eyes react to light, the ears to vibrations of air molecules, the nose to gaseous chemicals in the air, the tongue to chemical solutions and the skin to mechanical and temperature changes. Our range of susceptibility to each energy is also restricted. Light sensation provides a good example. The specialized neurones in the retina of the eye are excited by energies from only a small part of the electromagnetic spectrum. They do not respond to waveforms beyond the ultraviolet or infrared bands, only those in between. Similar limitations occur in our sensation of sound frequencies. Very high-pitched sounds and extremely low-pitched sounds are inaudible to human ears. Dogs and bats, however, can hear high frequencies inaudible to man.

A second limitation of the human sensory system is that there are some energies that we are unable to sense at all simply because we do not have sense organs that are sensitive to them. Magnetic waves and radio waves are examples of energies of which we are totally unaware, that is until they are converted by machines into energies that we are sensitive to (e.g. radio waves into sound). We still cannot, however, experience the waves in the air without mechanical assistance.

The transmission channel in the human perceptual system consists of sensory neurones, which travel from the sense organ to the area of appreciation in the brain. One sensory neurone carries information in the form of changes in electrical potential across the membrane of elongated fibres called axons. These cells can be inches or even more than 1 foot long. In this way information is carried from the sense organ to the area of appreciation in the brain in the form of electrical impulses travelling along several neurones. These impulses coming from the neurones are organized, co-ordinated and interpreted in the areas of appreciation in the brain to provide some internal representation of the external stimulus and its meaning.

The description of perception to this point suggests that processing is a one-way activity, information passing from the outside world to the brain where meaning becomes immediately apparent. Perception is not, however, a one-way process and much of our interpretation of external stimuli is a result of a guess-and-check mechanism sometimes called top-down processing (Boden, 1977). The decoding and interpretation of sensations depend on learning – the more we experience particular stimuli the better we are equipped to attaching meaning to them. Stimuli or sensations do not automatically carry meaning. Take for instance the symbol in Figure 2.5. The English reader will probably not attach specific meaning to this symbol in the same way that he may be able to attach a word to the symbol and yet there is still some compulsion to make the symbol meaningful.

One may suggest that it looks like a house, or even if the reader says that it is a Chinese symbol an interpretation has been made. Here the person is making the stimulus fit some idea that he or she has.

In a very subtle way, perception involves making a quick guess about the nature of the stimulus and then checking for features that support or reject the original guess. A simple experiment will confirm that the person's perception is influenced by factors arising in the area of appreciation as well as those from the outside world. Figure 2.6 shows two symbols. Show them to a friend and ask what numbers they are. The person is likely to say 10 and 13. If one asks another person what letters they are they are likely to say X and B. By telling the person what to look for, that is numbers or letters, we are imposing an expectation that influences the top-down process; this causes the interpretation to change while keeping the stimulus, and thus the bottom-up process, the same.

A relevance of the model of perception, described up to this point, to nursing can be summarized as follows:

1. Observation involves the collection of information in the form of external energy changes which are capable of being detected by sense organs.

Figure 2.5 A Chinese character.

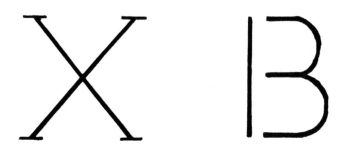

Figure 2.6 Ambiguous symbols.

2. Collection of information about our environment is limited because of the limitations of the sense organs.
3. Raw nervous impulses are organized, integrated and interpreted to produce meaning.
4. Interpretation of meaning depends on learning and experience.
5. Top-down processing suggests that human beings apply meaning to the stimulus rather than the stimulus automatically carrying meaning.

The most important implication for nursing observation is that the quality of observation depends on the nurses' knowledge, learning and experience. This will determine how they interpret the observed cues in the patient and his or her environment. The raw stimuli will be meaningless to nurses unless they can apply to them descriptive characteristics, object categories and possible consequences. Perception involves making guesses that, to a greater or lesser extent, are accurate reflections of the observer's outside world.

Attention

There are many thousand energy changes and features of the environment that the senses could detect in any one moment. The brain is not able to process all the information available, even to just one of the sense organs. If the reader of this book were to stop and make a list of every detail of his/her surroundings – colours, shapes, shades, movements, shadows and objects – then add to these all the sounds that can be heard with eyes closed, the taste and feeling inside the mouth, the feeling of touch and pressure on the surface of the body and the smells and feelings in the nasal cavity, an enormous list would be produced. Even so this would give only an inkling of the information available at any one time. The sensory apparatus must ignore some information while focusing on other if meaning is to be extracted from this barrage of information. This mechanism is commonly called 'attention', and the principle introduced here is that perception is selective.

If some features of the environment are excluded while others are picked up and processed, it is easy to suggest that there is some sort of filter to the potential sensory inputs. This has indeed been suggested (Broadbent, 1985), and it allows only a few sensory inputs to pass on to the organisational and interpretation centres of the perceptual system (Figure 2.7).

Attention not only involves selection of information in just one sensory modality; it is also achieved by closing down some sensations while concentrating on a difficult or interesting passage in a book. Similarly one is rarely aware of the pressure of clothing on the shoulders until attention is focused on this sensation.

Several things can influence this perceptual filtering process:

1. Needs of the observer. If someone is particularly hungry he or she will pay more attention to things that appear to be food.
2. Knowledge of the observer. We may pay little attention to a stimulus if we do not understand its meaning or importance. The nurse who does not realize the importance of a discoloration of a diabetic person's toe may not even notice it.
3. Interest and curiosity.
4. Tiredness or fatigue in the observer.
5. Sensory impairment. Damage to sense organs or nerves may interfere with ability to focus on particular aspects of the environment.
6. Expectations of the observer. This has already been demonstrated in the discussion of top-down processing.

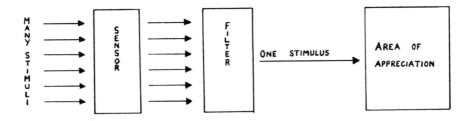

Figure 2.7 A model of perception including sensory filter.

7. Attitudes of the observer. Attitudes are relatively enduring predetermined thoughts, feelings and tendencies to action towards particular objects. They may affect the focusing ability of the perceptual system in much the same way as expectations.
8. Thought preoccupations and emotions of the observer.

All of these factors may influence the nurse's ability to make accurate observations. It is important to remember that the nurse must expend a certain amount of energy to attend to important features of the patient and ward off distractions arising from within herself and the environment. The effect of knowledge on attention once again demonstrates the importance of learning in improving the nurse's ability to select important information in the environment.

AREAS FOR NURSING OBSERVATION

The nurse is using these processes of perception to collect information about patients and the world that they live in. When observing patients' environments this can be their home or the surroundings they sees as their own (their territory) or the surroundings they finds themselves in. The patient's territory may just be the area surrounding his or her bed and locker, while in hospital. When observing the patient's environment the following points can be noted:

- tidiness and order
- cleanliness;
- temperature;
- noise;
- amount of light;
- appropriate use of objects;
- value of objects;
- state of repair of objects;
- hazards;
- amount of space;
- colours of surroundings;
- air pollutants/dust/smoke;
- personal possessions;
- luxuries;
- facilities.

The other object of observation will be the patient. Once again observation can be categorized under the three headings provided by the areas of human functioning: biological, psychological and social

(Table 2.4). The classification of observations into these categories is fairly arbitrary in that information in one area may provide information about problems in other areas. One example would be a biological observation of skin colour, that may yield information on some psychological state (e.g. blushing).

Observational Skill

To summarize, nursing observational skill involves:

1. Focusing attention on key stimuli in the environment.
2. Using knowledge and past experience to make interpretations about the meaning of stimuli.
3. Drawing up a patient-assessment *pro forma* that adopts the recommendations of one or more nursing models.
4. A consideration of all areas of human functioning in relatively equal proportions.

Table 2.4   Areas for Nursing Observation

Physiological	*Psychological*	*Social*
General appearance	Thought	Clothing
Skin colour	Feelings	Non-verbal cues
Skin damage	Ability to concentrate	Social involvement
Skin hygiene	Attitudes	Communicative style
Hair and nails	Memory	Friends
Mouth and teeth	Problem-solving	Family ties
Breathing	Level of consciousness	Affiliative needs
Cough	Reaction to pain	Roles
Sputum	Orientation	Class
Freedom of movement	Anxiety	Status around environment
Movement ability of limbs	Intellectual ability	Occupation, work
Unusual movement, involuntary movement	Ability to understand Beliefs	Financial status Educational background
Posture	Self-esteem	Language style
Form; contractures, deformity, swelling, lumps	Self-image Defence mechanisms Personality traits	Religious interests Social interests Group participation
Temperature	Motivations	Reaction to authority and
Pulse and apex beat	Needs	control
Blood pressure	Attention/awareness	Sexual behaviour
Urine	Creativity	Prejudices
Vomitus	Ability to learn	Social attitudes
Wound discharge	Likes and dislikes	Rapport
Faeces		
Sleep		
Eating habits		

5. Taking deliberate action to investigate features that are not immediately apparent.
6. Acting on observations made: e.g. reporting and taking remedial action.

REFLECTIVE ACTIVITIES

1. Take a piece of paper and list all the needs you feel that are most important to you. List them under the headings physiological, psychological and social.
2. The next time you are ill, for any reason, list the problems that you experienced as soon as you are well enough to do so.
3. Choose one patient whom you have been nursing for at least 1 week. List the patient's needs and problems (actual and potential) on the basis of the difficulties he or she is prepared to tell you about and your nursing knowledge. Place the patient's problems in order of priority.
4. Select a friend who is keen to co-operate in this activity. Both sit down and without discussion each draw up a list on a sheet of paper of the many ways in which you differ from each other. When you have finished compare each other's list. Make sure you choose somebody you know well and who knows you well.
5. In the room that you are sitting at the moment list everything you are aware of without moving. List each item under the following headings.
   (a) By sight only.
   (b) With eyes closed, only listening.
   (c) With eyes closed and without moving, all those things you can feel on your skin.
   (d) With eyes closed, all the smells you are aware of.
   (e) The taste in your mouth.
6. Ask three people to help you. Ask one to leave the room and plan to do something that lasts 5 mins when he or she returns. The remaining three then write down everything they observed about the 5 mins activity for as long as it takes afterwards. Now compare each other's notes.

SELF-EVALUATION TASKS

Do not read these until you are sure you understand this chapter.

1. Define the following terms: needs; potential problems; top-down processing; nursing observation.

2. List Roper's activities for daily living.
3. Describe in the shortest possible statements, what the major features are of three models of nursing.
4. Draw up a diagram to show the complex interrelationship between needs, problems, areas of human functioning and variation in human functioning.
5. List five activities that contribute towards observational skill.

Check your answers with the text.

CHAPTER 3

Communication skills

LEARNING OBJECTIVES

You should concentrate on being able to:

1. Define the word rapport.
2. Draw a diagram to show a human communications model.
3. List and briefly describe the human behaviours that transmit information under the headings verbal and non-verbal.
4. List seven functions of human communication.
5. List eight functions for nurse–patient communication.
6. List and briefly describe eight principles for sending a message effectively.
7. List and briefly describe four principles for receiving a message efficiently.
8. List the possible reasons for communication failure under the headings:
   (a) Encoding failures.
   (b) Transmission failures.
   (c) Channel failures.
   (d) Perceptual failures.
   (e) Decoding failures.
9. List principles for rectifying communication failures.
10. Give examples of the communicative attributes of each of the four areas of language study.
11. List seven methods of set induction for conversation.
12. List and briefly describe three methods of maintaining a conversation.
13. List and give examples of six groups of communicative error that relate to conversational skill.
14. Briefly describe five methods of set closure applicable to conversation.
15. Recall and use eight guidelines for communicating effectively in writing.
16. Describe and use eight principles for touching behaviour in nursing practice.

17. Define the term 'self-awareness'.
18. List three ways in which self-awareness can facilitate the performance of social skills.
19. List the types of information that may be obtained from interpersonal communication.
20. Define the terms interoception and introspection.

COMMUNICATION

If we accept that nursing is a relationship in which two people are involved in some transaction, we are encouraged to consider how human beings influence each other. Both parties share information, i.e. they both emit stimuli that are perceived by the other person, this other person acting on this information to maintain and mediate the interaction. Since the patient is often dependent on the nurse, the onus is on the nurse to become an efficient communicator. Communication skill is therefore essential to the nursing process. If the nurse wishes to carry out the nursing process efficiently and engage in social skills in an effective way she must become more **aware** of communication processes as they occur in real-life situations. This means consciously observing and analysing interpersonal communication rather than taking it for granted as is the usual habit. It has been pointed out that communication is carried out by all of us and that it is not therefore necessary to be taught something that is acquired naturally. Yet nursing, if it is to be a professional occupation, requires communication skills beyond those of the ordinary layman. This is particularly true in view of the fact that the patient is dependent on the nurse and patients often have difficulty participating in normal communication. The nurse should be able to plan a communication and analyse situations so that mistakes in communication are minimized, avoided or rectified. Communication is a human need and, as such, the nurse will need to become skilled in the art of helping patients to meet this need when they are unable to do so unaided. The relevance of communication may be demonstrated by the concept of rapport.

RAPPORT

A social skill often mentioned by nurses is 'gaining rapport' with the patient. This attitude is also encapsulated in phrases such as 'forming a relationship with the patient' and 'getting to know the patient'. Rapport describes a situation in which there is a mutual recognition and reciprocation of emotional state of each person when two people interact. In human relationships people share and act upon the feelings they have about each other. Each person's estimation of the effect he or she is having on the other person determines the depth and persistence of the subsequent interaction. There are various expressions people use to describe this situation, including 'getting along well together', 'love at first sight' and 'can't seem to hit it off'. They describe situations in which people are gaining or having difficulty gaining rapport.

Rapport depends upon each person sending out information to the other person about the feelings he or she has towards him or her. This interpretation of the feeling state of the other person is often a guess because the feelings are inferred from the person's behaviour. We can all recall mistakes in this area when we have thought that another person liked or disliked us and the converse was later found to be the case. When a person becomes aware of the feelings another person has towards him or her, he or she generally adjusts his or her behaviour to complement these feelings. Take for example a situation in which a person becomes bored by the conversation of another individual that he or she has just met. The 'boring' person, if he or she is able to realize this, must take action to rectify it if wishing to maintain the interaction. If the 'boring' individual does not notice his or her effect on the other person, or refuses to take rectifying action, the listener is likely to become frustrated and dissatisfied with this encounter. This is likely to result in a breaking off of any interaction and a reluctance by the frustrated person to repeat this unsavoury experience on future occasions. We can see that this activity of gaining rapport depends a great deal on each person's communicative ability and success or failure depends on the ability of each of the parties to reach some sort of shared understanding with the other. This process of maintaining interaction by recognizing and reciprocating the feelings of others is clearly of fundamental importance to the nursing relationship. It is very difficult to conceive of a helping relationship that does not involve constant interaction and mutual understanding. Nursing is by its very nature an intimate and shared experience that depends on an ability to achieve rapport.

WHAT IS COMMUNICATION?

Consider the following situations:

1. You call out to your dog 'sit' and he or she immediately does so.
2. A teacher walks into a noisy class, writes 'silence' on the blackboard and leaves without speaking. The pupils begin to whisper.
3. A female bee, after discovering a patch of flowers rich in nectar, returns to the hive, walks on the honeycomb among her fellows in a

ritual fashion. Minutes later the flowers are visited by many more bees.

4. A driver sees an amber, then a red light, and automatically steps on the brake.
5. You walk up to a person in a strange town to ask directions to the railway station. He looks away from you and continues to read a newspaper.
6. A man in a white coat walks into hospital to the operating theatre, changes into theatre clothing and watches an operation. He is not a doctor or any kind of medical person but leaves without being challenged.

What have all these diverse situations got in common? The answer is that they all involve processes in which meaning or information is passed from one source to another. Any changes observable in one object bringing about observable changes in another can be called communication. In the interpersonal context we would say that the objects of primary interest are two human beings. Which of the examples given above are examples of communication between people? Is a traffic light a means of communication between people?

The communication skills discussed in this chapter will be analysing communications, sending a message, receiving a message, communication fault-finding, speaking, conversation, writing and teaching skills.

ANALYSING COMMUNICATION

To be able to 'nurse' fellow human beings it is necessary to be able to bring to conscious awareness those events that allow communication to take place, to identify variations in communication and to be able to describe them. In this way nurses can understand more about their interactions with their patients and even describe them to the patients or teach others.

If nurses are to analyse communication they must have a mental image of a communications process, must be able to identify types of code and types of transmission methods, must understand the variation in message meaning and identify the function of individual communications.

A Communication Process

The approach described here is somewhat mechanistic but helps most efficiently to tease out elements suitable for analysis. This approach has been called information theory.

The four major elements in communication are: (i) the message;

(ii) the sender; (iii) the receiver; and (iv) the transmission channel. A message can be described as a set of symbols that carry information, i.e. some sort of agreed meaning. The message arises in the sender and is carried by some vehicle to the receiver. The process actually involves changes in the form of the information as it crystallizes in the sender, travels through the channel and is understood by the receiver. Imagine that a nurse sees that a patient is in danger from a falling brick. The process begins with a thought that the patient must move to avoid injury. The aim in communication here is almost to transfer this thought so that it becomes a thought experienced by the other person. The person must convert this thought into symbols that are capable of being carried by the transmission channel, in this case into words. The sounds of 'Watch out!' are emitted and travel through the air (transmission channel) to the endangered individual. The receiver, having special apparatus for sound reception (ears), collects the vibrations of the air (sound) and converts them to nervous impulses which cause patterns of neural activity in the brain. If the receiver is able to attach form to these 'noises', i.e. can appreciate that they are words (symbols), he or she may then be able to attach meaning to the words, then understanding that he or she must move to avoid some danger.

The process of converting the meaning into symbols is called *encoding* and the process of converting the symbol into meaning is called *decoding*. It is obviously important that both individuals share the same encoding and decoding procedure otherwise the communication would be useless. What would happen if the patient had no knowledge of the English language? It is interesting that the symbols 'watch out' vary in character from the original thought 'move to avoid injury'.

We can now construct a model that helps us to understand the communication process (Figure 3.1). It will be noticed that a pair of unusually named boxes have been added in the figure, the output selector and input selector. The former indicates a process by which symbols are transformed into nervous impulses, which in turn bring about some body movement that causes changes in the transmission

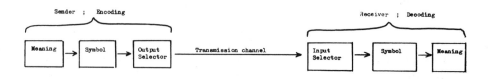

Figure 3.1 A communication model.

channel. These include the production of sound, smells, emission of light changes (movements) and heat. The input selector carries out the reception of a particular change in the environment (transmission channel), the conversion of these changes into nervous impulse and the activation of thought patterns. Input selectors help us to pay attention. This process from input to meaning is frequently termed 'perception'.

It will be useful to look at a different kind of communication in the same situation as described earlier. Imagine that the patient who hears 'Watch out' does not understand what is happening. The thought 'What's going on?' comes to mind. The thought may be encoded to cause a particular facial expression. This is transmitted as a pattern of light, which is received by the nurse whose eyes receive the light, converting it into nervous impulses and attaching meaning to it, i.e. 'He doesn't know what I'm saying'. While in this example the patient is now probably unconscious, it is obvious that communication is a two-way process and that each communicative act can generate another, in which case the sender becomes a receiver and the receiver a sender. It may also be apparent that much information can be transmitted in a variety of ways.

What Information Can Be Transmitted?

The simple answer to the question 'What can be communicated?' is 'Anything that has or carries meaning'. Some examples of the types of information that can be communicated can help us to understand the variety of such information. Perhaps the best way to begin is to take the example related earlier. Thoughts, ideas, beliefs or facts can be communicated. In the same way that the idea that a fellow human being must move can be placed in the consciousness of a fellow human being, other thoughts, facts or beliefs can also be communicated. In addition, emotions may also be communicated. Not only can somebody say he or she is happy, angry or miserable, he or she may look it or indicate it by tone of voice. Other aspects of human functioning such as intended behaviour or tendencies to action can also be communicated. When thoughts, emotions and tendencies to act are associated with one object and are predetermined almost in a reflex manner they are often called 'attitudes'. Many personal characteristics and traits, such as sex, age, abilities and habits may also be communicated to others. Information can also be transmitted about the person's social position; examples include class, status, occupation and role. Relationships between people and relationships between humankind and the environment are communicable. Other aspects about the person such as self-image and self-esteem can also be communicated to others.

Transmission of Information

According to the information theory approach, it has been suggested that the process of communication essentially involves encoding, i.e. changing meaning into a code or a system of symbols that have an agreed meaning. Information and meaning are much the same thing. The important feature is that both parties use symbols that have an agreed meaning otherwise they will carry no information. The symbols are transmitted by some form of human action (behaviour) to a fellow human being who is able to decode the message because of the shared system of meaning. It is worth considering now the ways in which transmission can be achieved. This is important because it is the only observable part of the communication process.

Two broad groups of human transmission behaviour are often described, **verbal** and **non-verbal**. Verbal communication involves the use of words (language) in either spoken or written forms. While verbal communication is dependent on vocal production behaviour, i.e. the use of laryngeal air vibration, mouth, tongue and pharyngeal shaping, not all vocal productions are verbal. One can identify a whole range of vocal sounds that humans can make that are not words but carry information. Examples include a scream or a baby's cry. Other aspects of oral sound production are communicative but are not verbal. Prosodic features such as intonation and stress fit into this communication category. How many ways can the sentence: 'I love you' be interpreted if one word is stressed or emphasized more than the others? How would the intonation (or tune) behind the words sound if declared in a tender moment or if phrased as a question?

The answers to these questions will demonstrate the importance of non-verbal vocal signals. Other non-verbal features include pitch, loudness and duration of sound. One can make the 'I love you' sentence change in meaning by saying it quickly or very slowly, in a deep voice or a high pitched voice, loudly or quietly. Argyle (1972) pointed towards other communicative channels in oral production. Features such as accent and voice quality have been called indexical features (Abercrombie, 1968) because they point to the speaker's personal characteristics. They do not add to the content of verbal communication but clearly transmit information. In Figure 3.2 the oral transmission channels mentioned here are summarized.

Non-verbal Transmission

Besides non-verbal aspects of speech, Argyle (1972) listed nine other non-verbal behaviours that transmit information, these comprise: (i) facial expression; (ii) head shaking and nodding; (iii) looking; (iv) gestures; (v) body contact and touch; (vi) appearance; (vii) proximity; (viii) orientation; and (ix) posture.

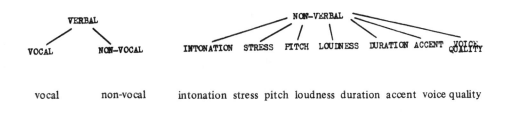

vocal   non-vocal   intonation stress pitch loudness duration accent voice quality

Figure 3.2 Oral transmission channels.

Facial Expression

We are all fully familiar with smiling, frowning and looks of surprise or fear. The face has been said to be the main second channel of communication used at the same time as speech (Argyle, 1969).

Head Shaking and Nodding

These have also been found to be fairly universal in communicating negative or positive orientations.

Looking

Eye contact and gaze are powerful communication channels. They are most powerful in indicating attention and looking away often controls turn-taking in conversation. Looking away has been found by Argyle to indicate that a person is about to speak, and a prolonged gaze indicates that he is about to finish. Eye contact also serves as a source of information about the listener, i.e. how he is receiving the information. Does he understand, does he believe it, does he find it funny, is he interested, etc.? Eye contact also provides a means of expressing emotions.

Gestures

Many examples of specific intentional limb movements convey information: hand-waving, shrugging shoulders, thumbs up, finger-pointing and beckoning, may all be familiar. The list of gestures used by different cultures is long (Morris, 1977).

Friedman and Hoffman (1967) suggested that gestures fall into two categories, those linked with speech and those that serve as tension releases. The former, they suggest, are intended as communicators but the latter are not.

Body Contact and Touch

much evidence to suggest that body contact is a basic animal ..eed (Harlow, 1959). Touch and physical contact are powerful ways of communicating emotion and relationships. They also provide a source of comfort. Infants often rush for body contact for relief from discomfort and unhappiness. Jourard (1966) discussed the significance of the different areas of the body that are touched and the variation in touching behaviour of the toucher. Where people touch each other and how often can indicate the relationship of the toucher and the touched and also the culture of both individuals (Figure 3.3).

One of the most noticeable functions of touch in adulthood is to

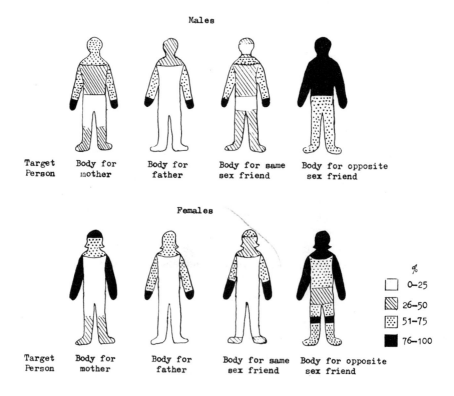

Figure 3.3 Interpersonal touching patterns – each figure shows percentage of people who reported being touched by the target person for different areas of the body. Source: adapted from Jourard (1966).

mark the degree of intimacy between two individuals. Sexual interest is indicated by an increase in touching behaviour, an increased acceptance of touching and a reciprocation of the touching behaviour. This provides an example of the way in which touch may carry emotional information to the participants and information about relationships to onlookers (Jones and Yarborough, 1985).

Appearance

Physical appearance may communicate many things; e.g. sex, age, state of hygiene and group membership. If one takes group membership as an example we may find many examples of how people indicate their membership of various groups – the bowler and pinstripes of the city businessman, the embroidered badge that shows membership of societies or institutions; the logo on the lapel, the tie or the teeshirt. Various youth cults have been identified by hairstyles – very long, extremely short, spiked and crew cut. From Cromwell's Roundheads to the 'Beatlecut' or even the 'punk fan', information about group membership has been conveyed by hairstyle. It is interesting that girls become intolerant of some hairstyles such as plaits and pony-tails as they become older. Wearing the clothing of an older age group is an attempt by many adolescents to communicate the predispositions of the age group they aspire to. Clothing must also fit the occasion or the individual may suffer extreme embarrassment. Body shape has been shown to cause greater concern in recent times with an increased interest in slimming in men as well as women. Uniforms are used for identification purposes, to instil fear as in the bearskin and red jacket of the Guards, or for practical purposes, in the case of protective clothing.

Sissons (1971) has shown the effect of physical appearance in communicating class position and the effect it has on interpersonal relationships. A person dressed in bowler hat, suit and umbrella receives different responses from passers-by when asking directions in comparison with the same person dressed in teeshirt, denim jacket and jeans.

Proximity

This is concerned with how close people come to each other during interaction. Argyle (1972) has suggested that people stand closer to those they like. It is interesting that in confined crowded spaces such as lifts or trains, strangers minimize eye contact when in unavoidably close proximity. There are considerable cross-cultural variations in tolerable proximity during interaction. Arabs and Latin Americans stand very close; Swedes, Scots and English stand much further apart.

Two people who begin sitting several tables apart move closer if verbal interaction is initiated and sustained. Distance tends to indicate aloofness or coldness, while close proximity suggests intimate relationships. Sometimes groups of three or four people stand so close during interaction that outsiders find it difficult to gain entry to the group. When somebody approaches another individual, for instance when a nurse walks towards a patient, much anticipation is experienced by that person ('what is she going to do to me?'). Pease (1984) suggested four main proximity zones depending on the purpose of the interaction. They are:

1. Intimate zone. Those who have an intimate relationship with each other will interact at a distance of approximately 18 inches.
2. Personal zone. Those who have a close personal relationship with other individuals will take up a distance of 18 inches to 4 feet.
3. Social/consultative zone. An appropriate distance for professionals to interact with their clients is 9–12 feet and it can often be from behind a desk.
4. Public zone. Speakers on public occasions are usually placed at a distance of 12 feet or greater from their audience.

It is useful to remember that even though the nurse–patient relationship may be seen as a professional–client relationship, nurses most often work in the intimate and personal zones. It is a useful exercise to consider how often nurses comes into the intimate zone (i.e. within 18 inches) of their patients.

Indeed the concept of territoriality, or personal space that one considers one's own, is of relevance here (Hayter, 1981). It can be disturbing for people if personal space is invaded. An area of 2 feet around a patient's bed and bedside locker could be viewed as his or her personal space. Any violation of that personal space can cause patients to feel at least uncomfortable and at most downright aggressive. Territoriality provides security, privacy, identity and autonomy for the owner of the space (Taylor, 1988). Hayter has described several factors that affect territoriality – such as age, sex, state of health and culture – and has considered the meeting of territoriality needs in nursing.

Argyle suggests that, in addition to indicating relationships, changes in proximity communicate the desire to initiate or terminate an encounter.

Orientation

Argyle describes this as 'the angle at which people sit or stand in relation to each other. The normal range is from head on (face-to-face) to side-by-side'. It has been found that friendly situations are characterised by side-by-side or right-angled arrangements. Face-to-face situations may be anxiety-provoking and may be seen as threatening or embarrassing (Pease, 1984). Orientation is closely related to proximity and eye contact (Wilkinson and Canter, 1982).

Posture

Two phrases from the *Oxford English Dictionary* (Simpson and Weiner, 1989) describe this form of communication aptly: 'To dispose the body or limbs of a person in a particular way . . . To pose for effect. . .'. Social power relationships may be demonstrated by posture. Argyle (1972) describes the superior (or dominant) posture, which consists of standing erect, with head tilted back and sometimes hands placed on hips. Can the reader remember seeing a ward sister in this position? Inferior (or submissive) posture involves a slight cower to look smaller, arching of the shoulders and a bowing head. A communication of attention by posture bears particular relevance to some of the skills described in this book. In the sitting position, when paying attention or showing lively participation, people tend to sit forward. Disinterest is communicated by sitting back almost in a slouched position. Open posture indicates an unguarded attitude, that we are not fearful or inhibited. The closed posture, with arms folded, folded leg position (ankle on knee of other leg) and curling into a ball, indicates that barriers are being formed with the intention of the person being guarded and defensive. Postural echo (Figure 3.4) is an interesting phenomenon that indicates a degree of genuine friendship or strong rapport between two people. The two individuals act as mirrors to each other's posture. Morris (1977) says that the attitude being expressed is 'see, I am just like you' and it demonstrates equality in a relationship. If the reader looks for postural echo in day-to-day interaction it can result in such amusement that it can be difficult to be sensible in interactions with others. It is difficult and embarrassing to accept that we seem to be copying each other, although this is probably because we do it unconsciously.

The Functions of Communication

It is useful in analysing communication to be able to identify the various uses to which it may be put. In order to do this one must be armed with a checklist of possible functions. R. Stevens (1975) describes eight functions of communication, which will serve to guide this discussion.

Communication may be used in order to achieve some gain, i.e. meet some need. When a patient asks for something to relieve pain, a bedpan, or for a 'date', the communication is primarily **instrumental**.

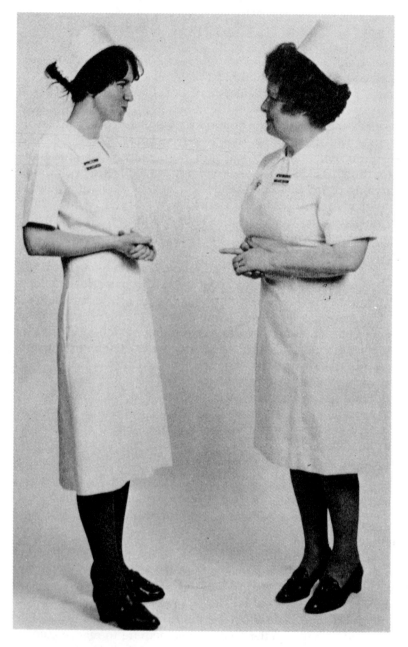

Figure 3.4 Postural echo.

The patient who asks questions wants to gain information. The nurse who fills in a time card or writes an essay in an examination is engaging in some instrumental communication. A second function is the **control** function, i.e. getting other people to do things. Nurses often say that they encourage patients to do deep-breathing exercises or persuade them to stop smoking. Nurses 'ask' the patient to remain in bed, remove his clothes, roll over for an injection and take his medication. We physically lift patients into sitting positions in bed or roll them over while a bed bath is being carried out. In many ways too numerous to mention nurses attempt to control patients. Perhaps the reader can think of ways in which patients control nurses?

Communication may also serve an **information** function, i.e. to transmit ideas, facts and cognitions. Libraries are information retrieval centres using various communication media. Information booklets in hospital and answers to questions from patients are examples of this function. However, when the doctor shakes his head when viewing a patient's radiograph or the nurse looks startled when asked by a patient 'Am I going to die?', information is also gleaned by the patient. The nurse did not mean to provide information but pointed to another function of communication, to express feeling. The **expression** function is generally facial. Patients can indicate pain, anxiety, depression, aggression, joy, or dislike of the nurse without saying a word. Yet often we also actually describe or try to describe how we feel. Communication can be used in the service of self-expression in many other ways by indicating class, group membership, attitudes and occupation. Nurse or doctors may wish to emphasize their medical background by using technical jargon, sometimes deliberately. Patients may make various attempts to use their own occupational jargon when personal identity is being threatened. Patients also express attitudes about the staff and hospital to relations and others. Communication may also be used just to maintain contact with other human beings. Much communication controls and regulates human encounters (Argyle, 1972). Discussion about the weather and other superficial chit-chat may often serve the function of facilitating contact.

It has been shown that medical personnel in intimate social encounters use quite sophisticated methods to make the social contact bearable. An example of this is the elimination of sexual connotation in the gynaecological examination (Emerson, 1970). Often people withdraw from others when depressed. They can find it difficult to initiate human contact and maintain it. An example occurs in the disorder schizophrenia, which is characterized by lack of intentional or appropriate communication. People often communicate more with others when anxious, and the function of communication in the **alleviation** of stress is well documented (Scheier *et al.*, 1986; Baron,

1989). The nurse's ability to reassure a patient is dependent on skills rooted in communication techniques. Sometimes patients, particularly those isolated in a single room, use the call alarm particularly often, for trivial things. This may serve a social contact function but it may also relieve boredom. It has often been said that one of the advantages of the old Nightingale Ward, in which 20 or so patients were housed in one large room, was that patients were kept stimulated by constant activity. This indicates that communication can also have a **stimulation** function.

The last function of communication described by R. Stevens (1985) has been called **role-related** or **ritual** function. Much communication may be determined by the situation in which we find ourselves. Indeed, one criticism of many nursing procedures and interactions is that nurses involve themselves in too much behaviour that is stereotyped. This is betrayed in phrases such as 'Won't be long now', 'How are we today then?', 'This may hurt a little', 'This will be cold', 'Everything will be alright', 'Try and keep still', 'Just lift up', 'Roll over', 'I've come to give you your injection'. It is common to hear interactions between nurse and patient totally determined by role. Being brave, communicating pain subtly, being subservient, talking about bowels and waterworks, may all be seen as appropriate to the patient role, while arguing with diagnosis, talking about football or a hole in the patient's sock may not.

These analyses of the functions of communication are very general and sociologically based. It may be useful, therefore, to examine the particular functions that communication may serve in the context of nursing.

Aims of Nurse–Patient Communication

Ashworth (1980) suggested four aims of nurse–patient communication. It may be useful to try to decide which of the functions described by R. Stevens coincide with each of the aims described here:

1. To establish a relationship in which the patient perceives the nurse as friendly, helpful, competent and reliable, and as recognizing the patient's worth and individuality (i.e. social contact, information function, expression).
2. To try to determine patients' needs as perceived by them, and when necessary, to help them recognize their other needs as perceived by the nurse (i.e. information functions, possibly role-related)
3. To provide factual information on which patients can structure their expectations (information).
4. To assist patients to use their own resources and those offered to

them (e.g. information) to meet their own needs (stimulation and control functions?).

Communication can serve instrumental functions in nursing. Some obvious examples include asking for help or for something to be obtained. Other examples are not so obvious, one being the achievement of recovery. In two important studies Hayward (1975) and Boore (1978) indicated that communication can reduce postoperative pain and anxiety and promote the patient's recovery. The expression function of communication may be demonstrated when the nurse attempts to maintain the patient's personal identity. Ashworth makes interesting observations on this issue in her research on communication in the intensive care unit:

> One way to maintain the patient's personal identity is discussion of his or her home, personal interests or other things connected with his daily life before admission to hospital. It may seem surprising that communication of this kind (category B) constituted only 3–7% of the total verbal communication to patients since 89% of the staff listed it as something they would include when talking to patients.
>
> *Ashworth, 1980*

The establishing of nurse–patient relationships involves, to a great extent, the allowing of personal expression. It is possible to consider in this context the aim of maintaining equality in the nurse–patient relationship. It is not uncommon to hear the following comment/response/dialogue in nurse–patient relationships:

Patient	Nurse
It hurts	No it doesn't
I'm frightened	Don't be silly
I want to go to the toilet	No you don't
I'm going to be sick	No you're not

This sequence reveals the persistence of nurse-centred relationships. The 'nurse knows best' phenomenon is taken to the limit here, although it is obvious that this is often not the case. Many a fouled bed or nurse's uniform has resulted from the last two instances given above and perhaps worse consequences may result from the first two. If nursing is to be patient-centred, personalized and the patient is to be treated as a human being – as an equal contributor to his or her own recovery (when possible) it is necessary to eliminate unnecessary subordinating aspects of the patient's role. Communication skills can help to achieve more interpersonal equality between nurse and patient (Bridge and Macleod Clark, 1981).

To summarize, the functions by which communication can serve the nurse may be:

- to establish and maintain a relationship with the patient;
- to promote the equality of the relationship;
- to collect information about the patient;
- to give information to the patient;
- to allow the patient self-expression;
- to promote recovery;
- to reassure the patient;
- to control the patient's and other people's behaviour.

SENDING A MESSAGE EFFICIENTLY

When sending a message it is necessary for the nurse to realize how important it is to be efficient. The consequences of inaccuracy or non-reception should be assessed. What will happen? Will the patient be harmed or become unhappy? Will rapport be lost? Will the patient become lost, confused or misguided?

To send a message efficiently one can adopt a method in keeping with the information theory model described earlier. The first phase involves the crystallization of the meaning of the information to be sent. This will involve stopping for a moment to become consciously aware of what is to be communicated – a classical situation of 'think before you act'. We are dealing here with intentional message communication, which assumes that the message can be brought to conscious awareness. Often people send messages unintentionally, as in the case of some non-verbal communications. This, however, does not mean that non-verbal channels cannot be used intentionally. Actors develop this skill to the full.

The second phase in sending a message will involve choosing a code. The code will be a spoken or non-verbal symbol. The appropriate mode must also be chosen. This may be permanent as in the case of written languages and sound-recorded speech, or transient as in the case of spoken and non-verbal communications. In the case of permanent forms, it is possible to carry out the encoding activity by either recording the message or writing it out, in order to assess the efficiency of the message. This brings up an important requirement in the sending of messages – the receiving of feedback. As a general rule it can be said that the more one seeks feedback, the more skilled one can become in spontaneous message emission. Examples include delivering speeches and giving explanations or instructions.

As mentioned previously, non-verbal communication can be improved by receiving feedback by frequent practice. A familiar example in nursing is smiling in the face of revulsion when the patient fouls the bed or has a particularly necrotic wound. The nurse can learn to do this relatively easily. An additional attribute of feedback is that it tells us about message reception, not just emission behaviour. One should always check with the person who receives the message that he has received the meaning correctly. It may be necessary to reformulate the code, choose another transmission channel or select a different behaviour to transmit the intended meaning. The sender may need to support the main transmission channel with other channels to ensure accuracy of the message. Telephone messages, written reports and sound-recorded messages often need precision because supporting channels are absent or limited.

The nurse should actively use checking behaviour because it is often the case that patients may not let the nurse know if they have understood the message. As a charge nurse, this author often had to go back to patients after the consultant's rounds to explain to them what he had said or what he meant. The doctor gave a very clear message but his accent, the terminology he used, patient anxiety or distractions by members of the assembled company often interfered with the message. Checking may be achieved by asking the patient to repeat the message in his or her own words or, in the case of non-verbal cues, asking the other person how he or she interpreted them. The whole process of sending messages involves paying attention to your own sending behaviour and the other person's response to this behaviour.

So to send an efficient message:

- assess the consequences of inaccuracy;
- carefully consider what the meaning will be;
- choose a code consciously;
- capture the attention of the receiver;
- select the transmission behaviour consciously;
- pay attention to one's own behaviour;
- pay attention to the receiver's response;
- check the receiver's interpretation of the message.

This can be tried when using the telephone.

RECEIVING A MESSAGE EFFICIENTLY

It is the responsibility of the professional nurse to take the initiative when receiving as well as when sending messages. The first stage in receiving is paying attention to the behaviour of the sender, in particular those behaviours directly concerned with the communication of the message. A problem the receiver can experience is that he may not be paying attention to the correct transmission channel or it may be so quick, as in the case of a 'wink', that the receiver may miss the cue completely. Occasionally the beginning of a message may be missed, while the receiver is trying to latch onto the channel being used. The nurse in this situation may need to ask the sender to begin again or repeat the message, especially when the communication is important. Notice that this involves paying attention to all transmission channels, not just speech and sound.

Receiving messages will involve encouraging the sender to communicate freely. This involves giving various rewards (reinforcements) such as social approval, attention or enthusiasm; certain attributes such as patience and tolerance can also facilitate communication.

The next phase of the receiving process involves giving feedback, i.e. cues that indicate whether the message is being understood or not. The receiver controls the quality of the message in this way and may need to exaggerate or use non-verbal and verbal cues for this purpose, practice again making perfection possible. One can actually provide feedback by saying that part of the message has not been understood or one can ask for repetition, e.g. 'Can you say that again?', 'Did you frown?' When answering a telephone or listening to a long telephone conversation (if ethical and possible) one can experience feedback principles being employed by listening to the number of checking comments that are made. One can consider why it is useful to give name, role and department when answering the telephone. How do we manage in this situation to cope with the absence of non-vocal/ non-verbal cues? This sort of observation can reveal the importance of feedback in message reception.

A final point about message receiving is also related to feedback. This concerns checking the 'meaning' of the message. While we expect words to mean the same thing to all who use the language, sometimes we do not interpret words properly when we infer their meaning. Sentences can be ambiguous, as can facial expressions and many non-verbal cues. If somebody raises an open hand, does it mean a friendly greeting or should one expect a slap on the face? Receiving messages involves checking and feeding back meaning. This may be achieved by questioning, reflecting, summarizing and paraphrasing.

To summarize, receiving a message involves:

- paying attention using all senses;
- encouraging and rewarding the sender;
- giving feedback;
- checking that the meaning has been accurately interpreted.

SET INDUCTION

An important sub-skill relevant to sending and receiving messages is set induction (Hargie *et al.*, 1981). This involves creating the right climate for the other person to give or receive messages. A whole series of actions may get the person ready to give or receive messages. Set induction involves setting the scene, preparing for action or gaining attention. Set induction will be discussed in greater detail in the sections on conversational and interviewing skills.

COMMUNICATION FAULT-FINDING

Communication failure in interpersonal transactions can cause many problems. These breakdowns can be the cause of such misunderstanding that people can be brought into conflict with each other. In a professional nursing sense, communication failure can cause confusions that have dangerous consequences. At other times, nurses may have difficulty in helping their patients because of the patients' inability to participate in interpersonal communication in their usual way. One of the key functions of the nurse is to help the patient to communicate when this ability is interfered with. The skill of communication fault-finding is suggested as a social skill for nursing simply because the consequences of poor interpersonal communication in health care can be disastrous. In addition, many other social skills depend, to a certain extent, on an ability to realize when there are communication problems and to identify the particular causes. There are several ways in which barriers to effective communication can be described (Douglass, 1992). In the context of the information theory model already described, one can group problems under five headings: (i) encoding failures; (ii) transmission failures; (iii) channel interference; (iv) perceptual failures; and (v) decoding failures.

Encoding Failures

Several problems can occur in the thought processes that begin the sequence of communication events. Perhaps the simplest cause is an impairment of brain functioning, e.g. with unconsciousness, stupor and delirium. Memory impairment, such as occurs in old age, can diminish the ability to select appropriate words or non-verbal cues. Confused thought, as experienced in some mental disorders, may cause encoding problems. Schizophrenia provides examples of this when neologisms, word salad, thought blocking and 'knights move' (sideways thinking) cause severe communication difficulties. Understanding of a language and ability to use it may influence communication in that the partner in communication may not share the encoding strategy employed. Limited vocabulary, restrictive code (see following discussion and Bernstein, 1959), the less developed language of children and second language learning may all cause encoding communication difficulties. In all these situations people cannot 'express themselves' clearly enough. A final example of encoding failure is caused by emotional factors. Severe emotions such as anxiety or aggression may make it difficult for people to encode in exactly the way they want. We can all find it difficult to express the meaning we want while having arguments. Sometimes we say things spontaneously, things we do not mean, and pick wrong words and even phrases and sentences in the 'heat of the moment'.

Transmission Failure

Even when the person has decided upon a message, the problem may originate in his or her inability to choose the transmission mode and in the use of that particular mode. Paralysis of various parts of the body can interfere with communicative ability. Gestures may be impossible when arms are paralysed and facial expression alters when hemiplegia has occurred; similarly, speech is difficult with facial paralysis. Problems may arise from uncontrollable body movements such as a twitch, tremor, squint, exophthalmos, stutter and risus sardonicus. Another factor that may interfere with message emission is impaired consciousness. Drugs or poisons may cause motor inability, slurred speech being a good example. Some physical and psychological disabilities may cause people to be mute. Some are constitutional in that the person has never been able to speak, while others may be induced as in the case of glossectomy and laryngectomy. The orthodontist can wire a person's jaw together, or in other conditions of oral surgery the mouth may be packed with dressing material or tubing. Severe dyspnoea can make speech difficult; sometimes severe emotional shock causes the person to become mute as a result of a hysterical reaction. It will also be obvious that fear and anxiety may inhibit message transmission. Imagine the effect of being told you will be shot if you speak!

A final example of a transmission problem is when the person absolutely refuses to transmit messages, thoughts or ideas. Negativism and resistance provide examples of this.

Channel Interference

Once the message has been transmitted the symbols may be distorted in several ways. Overload can be one cause of interference; this may be channel overload or attention overload. Sometimes the mode of transmission (the channel) may cause some complication – i.e. when two people speak at once or when somebody speaks too quickly.

Another example is gestures. Hand signals, such as signals for the deaf, can be too rapid for the novice user. Attention overload really involves competition for the receiver's attention. So many stimuli may be present that the different senses are confused.

The reader may be familiar with the situation in which several communications interfere with reception of one of them. Try switching on the radio, watching the television and moulding some plasticine into a star shape while listening to a person explain something that is fairly complicated. There is evidence that we can close down various sensory inputs to pay attention to one in particular but we can still be distracted by stimuli impinging on other senses. 'Noise' is a concept from information theory, which describes a form of interference concerned with competition for a particular sense. Examples of noise include the crackling or humming on the telephone that may make it difficult to hear what a person is saying. Noise, in fact, consists of meaningless stimuli that break up the message stimulus because the noise stimulus is similar to the message stimulus. 'Noise' is not restricted to sound channels. Visual examples include searching for a polar bear in a snow storm or looking for a coloured bead on a heavily patterned carpet.

A final problem loosely connected with channel interference is the relative permanence of the communication medium. One of the characteristics of speech is that each cue (i.e. sound, letter, word, phrase) fades away. The receiver must then resort to memory to keep track of the message and even if repeated the cues are never exactly the same. Other forms of communication may be permanent, allowing the receiver to go back over the same cues, obvious examples being the written word or the diagram. Photographs and films may permanently record non-verbal cues. The slow-action replay uses this advantage of permanent communication to the full. Problems in transmission can occur when messages are not in permanent form and human memory is the only form of permanence.

Perceptual Failure

This refers to an impairment in the person's ability to receive particular sensory stimuli. The blind and partially blind have visual reception problems, the deaf and partially deaf have auditory communication problems. Some other causes of visual and auditory sensory impairment include illusions and hallucinations. Treatment for diseases of the eyes or ears may involve them being covered by a dressing or medication, thus impairing function. Some diseases interfere with the ability of the eyes to accommodate to light or distance, or they may become too sensitive to light. Tinnitus is a condition that interferes with auditory perception by causing ringing in the ears. Loss of touch sensation in the condition of paraesthesia or anaesthesia would result in the inability to deal with any communication involving touch. Drugs may act on the nervous system to interfere with perception (e.g. to give blurred vision). The most severe sensory impairment is unconsciousness; however, it should never be forgotten that, when regaining consciousness, sometimes auditory sensation returns before motor ability. This is why nurses should be careful about the content of their conversations near unconscious persons and should always talk to the unconscious person just in case he or she can hear.

Decoding Failure

Making sense of the message or changing the code into meaning can be interfered with in several ways. The receiver may not share the same code conventions as the sender. Language difference provides an example of a person being unable to decode a message from another person. Languages do not even have to be totally different – sometimes dialect can make the message incomprehensible. Many people have been confronted with English dialects that they find impossible to understand.

Non-verbal communication modes also depend on agreed meanings. Different cultures interpret gestures differently, e.g. tapping the nose with one finger has different meanings in Italy and England (Morris, 1977). Cultural differences may also account for incongruity in thinking style or habit. Eskimos have many forms of the word 'snow', while English has only a few. It is extremely difficult to communicate the idea of space travel to a person of some equatorial tribe if he or she has no concept of outer space, the aeroplane or fuel energy. Less extreme forms of incongruity in thinking habits may also make decoding difficult. Technical terminology and jargon cause decoding difficulties for the person who has not learned the particular convention (e.g. with patients and medical jargon). One of the reasons children make decoding mistakes is because of their poorly developed vocabulary. A baby may call an aeroplane 'birdie' because he or she has associated the word with all things moving in the sky. The baby must learn to discriminate between 'birdie' and aeroplane.

Some disorders of thinking capacity also cause decoding problems. Delusions may cause the mentally ill to misinterpret information or cues from other people. Friendliness cues may be seen as deceptions to cause harm. Sometimes the deluded person believes that others are talking in a special code, meaning other things to those indicated in their utterances. Suspicion can cause even those who are well to misinterpret what others say or do. Certain expectations and attitudes, particularly prejudice, held by the receiver can interfere with decoding. Finally impairment of nervous functioning such as in confusion, tiredness or drug treatment may cause communication difficulty by interfering with decoding ability.

The elderly provide a good example of the possible complexity of communication failure that the nurse may encounter. Pauline Fielding (Bridge and Macleod Clark, 1981) gives an excellent insight into this situation by describing problems such as poor hearing, poor eyesight, speech difficulties, pain, fatigue, tiredness and confusion, which can cause faults in communication between the nurse and the elderly patient.

Remedial Action

The ability of the nurse to **identify** the cause of the communication failure is not sufficient on its own. Nurses must be able to take action in an attempt to rectify or minimize the fault whether it be found in themselves or others, in the sender or receiver. The following checklist is a suggested general approach to the remedial action that can be taken:

1. Simplify the message. This involves cutting out irrelevant cues (e.g. words) and may even mean resorting to single word communication (Ley, 1988). Telegraphic speech provides a good example of sentence simplification (Brown, 1976).
2. Strengthen the stimulus. Mechanical means for doing this, such as hearing aids and spectacles, are common. When one shouts to a deaf person one is adopting this policy of strengthening the stimulus. Cutting down 'noise' and interference will also facilitate this action. Do not confuse channels, as occurs when people shout at the blind.
3. Change channel. If a person cannot hear, use sign language or write down the message. Some hospitals have ready prepared symbol cards for nurses to communicate with the deaf and *vice versa*. Figure 3.5 shows a compilation of signs for common needs and instructions occurring in hospital. It is also worth remembering that lip reading is a language body movement channel to the deaf. Those with sight impairment will need to hear rather than read, and touch also becomes an important communication channel for such people.
4. Give feedback. Help the person to realize the cause of communication failure. This may allow the sender or receiver to assist in taking action. A person of a different language may suggest a friend who can interpret. The person may stop using vague or confusing signals.
5. Give support. Reinforcement, patience and encouragement will be

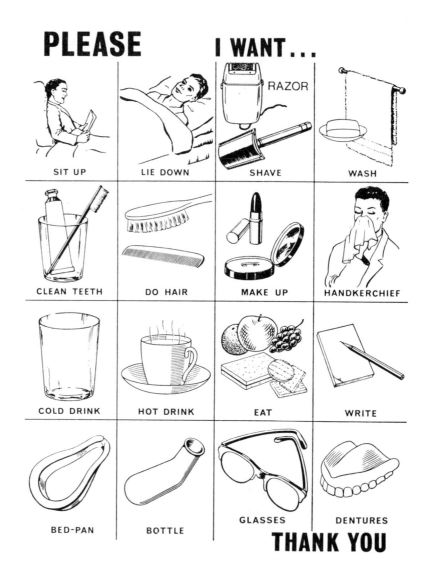

PLEASE **I WANT...**

SIT UP	LIE DOWN	SHAVE (RAZOR)	WASH
CLEAN TEETH	DO HAIR	MAKE UP	HANDKERCHIEF
COLD DRINK	HOT DRINK	EAT	WRITE
BED-PAN	BOTTLE	GLASSES	DENTURES

THANK YOU

Figure 3.5 Symbol card to assist communication in hospital. Source: The Chest, Heart and Stroke Association, with permission. The chart may be obtained from the Association at Tavistock House North, Tavistock Square, London WC1H on receipt of £2.00 to cover the cost of the chart and postage.

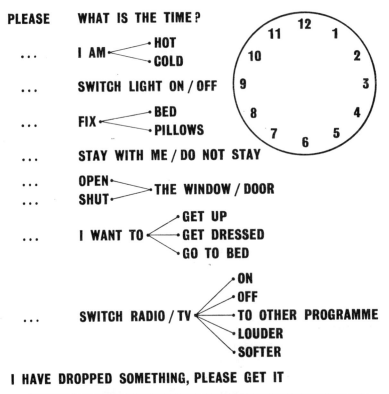

PLEASE   WHAT IS THE TIME ?

...   I AM →· HOT
                  ·→ COLD

...   SWITCH LIGHT ON / OFF

...   FIX →· BED
                  ·→ PILLOWS

...   STAY WITH ME / DO NOT STAY

...   OPEN·
...   SHUT·→ THE WINDOW / DOOR

...   I WANT TO →· GET UP
                        · GET DRESSED
                        · GO TO BED

...   SWITCH RADIO / TV →· ON
                                · OFF
                                · TO OTHER PROGRAMME
                                · LOUDER
                                · SOFTER

I HAVE DROPPED SOMETHING, PLEASE GET IT

A	B	C	D		
E	F	G	H		
I	J	K	L	M	N
O	P	Q	R	S	T
U	V	W	X	Y	Z

necessary to prevent frustration in those who have difficulty in understanding and being understood.
6. Remove causes of communication failure wherever possible. Disease, interference or threat, once eliminated, may alleviate communication failures.

A useful description of the planning of nursing care to cope with communication problems is given in Borsig and Steinacker (1982). They discuss several communication problems that may be encountered in the intensive care unit.

LANGUAGE SKILLS

Language is social skill simply because it involves at least two people, e.g. the nurse and the patient, in a shared activity. It is one of the major forms of human communication and is significant because it is one of the features that clearly distinguishes humankind from animals. Not only does language allow communication, it also provides the basic symbolic representations involved in most of our thoughts. Language may influence thought so much that Whorf (1952, 1956) has suggested that people around the world 'see' the world in different ways. Language can dictate the form in which we create the symbols and images that represent our world in our thoughts.

The importance of language skills in nursing practice has been demonstrated by the amount of nursing research on verbal communication (see Wilson-Barnett, in Bridge and Macleod Clark, 1981). Kron (1972) suggests three language skills are necessary for nursing; these are speaking, writing and reading. Speaking is universally used by people, whereas writing and reading depend on education and social need. All three skills take on added importance in nursing when one considers that efficiency in practising these skills has implications for the standards of patient care.

SPEAKING

In order to understand better the speaking skill, it is useful to look at the distinctive properties of human speech. Hockett (1960, 1963) and Hockett and Altman (1968) describe 16 distinctive features of speech:

1. Vocal-auditory channel. Voice production and ear reception.
2. Broadcast transmission (heard by all in the vicinity not just restricted to one person) and directional reception (we can spot who is speaking very easily, the origin of the speech can be located).

3. Rapid fading. Spoken words are not permanent stimuli.
4. Interchangeability. Here the speaker and listener can perform the same functions. One person can repeat the other's spoken phrases.
5. Total feedback. Here a person can hear his or her own speech as well as others.
6. Specialization. The essential function of speech is communication.
7. Semanticity. It can carry sophisticated, relatively precise meaning compared with other communication modes.
8. Arbitrariness. Meaning is arbitrary, allowing a high degree of flexibility and limitless range of possible communication topics.
9. Discreteness. Speech meaning is communicated by very precise sounds. Minor differences change meaning radically. It is discrete not continuous.
10. Displacement. Can refer to things not physically present in time or space. Refers to past, future and things not visible.
11. Openness. The capacity to say things that have never been said or heard before, which can be understood by other language users.
12. Transmission. Passed on from one generation to another.
13. Duality of patterning. The meaning is carried by the pattern of sounds not the sounds themselves, at two levels, variety of words (sound patterns) and word combinations.
14. Prevarication. Can be used to lie, talk nonsense or deceive.
15. Reflexiveness. Language can be used to describe itself.
16. Learnability. Here the speaker of one language can learn others.

Speaking to others involves using a communication mode that has all of these features. It is possible now to summarize by giving guidelines for effective speech drawn from the points made above concerning characteristics of language and speech.

Deliberate, professional, effective speech requires preparation. Where speaking serves vital functions the nurse must, to quote the old adage, 'think before he or she speaks'. In some situations, such as public speaking, one may need to write down what is to be said in order to aid efficient smooth delivery. Prior thought may involve decisions concerning content and grammar form (phrase structure). Those nurses who habitually use restricted code may need to concentrate on efficient elaborated code formulation. On other occasions, they **may** need to formulate restricted code to aid patient communication. We have seen that the person using restricted code understands elaborated code fairly well but may find an elaborated code cold and clinical because he or she sees restricted code as an indicator of social intimacy and friendliness. Elaborated code may have a distancing effect.

Once one has formulated the form of the utterance, it may be necessary to secure and maintain the attention of the listener. The nurse should pay attention to her speech production because of the effects of articulation on word and phrase meaning. Control of pauses between phonemes and words will assist articulation and the use of pauses between phrases can prove to be a particularly effective ploy. Pauses allow time to think, reflect and rest. The use of tone and inflection may prevent monotonous speaking and help to emphasize the important words and topics that are being presented. Many of these features carry indexical meaning and they will communicate much about the nurse's personal attributes, professional ability and attitude to the patient. Volume is of particular importance. Speaking too quietly in one-to-one communication may frustrate the other person or indicate lack of confidence; if speech is too loud, one may seem to be aggressive or dominant.

When speaking to groups of people one must use broadcast transmission to the full, learning to speak adequately even when one is compelled to increase speech volume or project utterances some distance. Talking for the sake of talking is rarely satisfying for the listener, even though it can be pleasing to the speaker. Economy of words while maintaining clarity of meaning is a professional skill that has many advantages in nursing and any occupation in which time is at a premium. Speech imperfections and distracting habits should be minimized. Some non-communicative vocal habits are distracting and many are unnoticed. It is common to hear others say 'Er', during speech pauses, or use redundant phrases such as 'Do you know what I mean?' Most of us do not notice the frequency with which we and others have these speech habits, until we focus on them. Such habits should be minimized when they interfere sufficiently enough with language production that it makes comprehension difficult for the listener. Efficient nurse speakers should actively receive feedback to assess the effects of her vocalizations on others. Differences in language use between oneself and the listener should be identified at an early stage, so that appropriate modifications can be made. These variations may be due to the stage of language development, total inability to use or understand the language, dialect or elaborated/restricted code.

CONVERSATION

The importance of conversation and time for one-to-one contact between the nurse and patient has been emphasized by many nurse researchers (e.g. Wilson-Barnett, in Bridge and Macleod Clark, 1981). Conversation will be taken to mean a relatively informal exchange of speech on a one-to-one or small-group basis. The general function of conversation is to maintain social contact and provide shared sensory stimuli. While many forms of communication may be observed during human conversation, it will be presumed here that the emphasis is upon shared speech. Conversational skill can be examined in three stages – set induction, maintaining conversation and set closure.

The term set induction has been discussed by Hargie *et al.* (1981). It is the process of entering into social interaction, the beginning of social contact. Beginning interaction involves securing attention, making initial contact, setting the scene, preparing for action and adopting positions and orientations which facilitate the interpersonal transactions which will take place.

Set Induction for Conversation

Hargie *et al.* (1981) indicate several actions that may be used to induce set for conversation, these are: (i) using novel stimuli; (ii) posing an intriguing problem; (iii) making provocative statements; (iv) unusual behaviour; (v) non-threatening initial approach behaviour; (vi) facilitative comment; and (vii) providing 'creature comforts'.

Using novel stimuli

One can present newspaper headlines, photographs or diagrams in order to begin conversations in the hope that they will elicit conversation. The nurse who wears a tabard decorated with a familiar character may encourage a child to enter into discussion, as may the presentation of a new toy.

Posing an intriguing problem

This provokes thought and attention, either by arousing interest or curiosity. Patients would commonly capture a nurse's attention by saying 'I have this problem, which I have not mentioned to anybody'. Sharing a problem is often flattering and it is a privilege but it generally arouses our curiosity.

Making a controversial or provocative statement

This, of course, should be done without offending the other person. Statements that are emotive, value-ridden and that are difficult to conclude by acceptable responses or identifying single correct answers are particularly suitable for this purpose.

Carrying out unusual or unexpected behaviour

Careful thought will be required here by the nurse. Role expectations and institutional constraints can limit the nurse's use of this method of set induction. The seriousness of many patients' problems is inconsistent with any tendency to flippancy. The imaginative nurse may find times when she may engage in this method of set induction in an acceptable and appropriate way. An important point to remember is that if the nurse engages in any behaviour that is unusual or unexpected, such as walking up to the patient with a fully equipped trolley, suddenly acting suspiciously or not talking to the patient, she may be drawn into conversations because her behaviour provides stimulus to the patient. Strange behaviour resulting from the instruction 'Do not tell Mr Smith about his terminal condition', may in this way draw the nurse into situations where the patient probes to find out what is wrong.

Non-threatening initial approach behaviour

Smiling, being polite, non-threatening and putting the person at ease, all help when initial contact is made. One may shake hands or give facial cues (e.g. eyebrow flash) to indicate recognition of the other person (Morris, 1977).

Facilitative comment (non-task comment)

Comments such as 'How are you?' or 'Hello, nice to see you' help to bring about interaction. One may make flattering comments about appearance or dress, or ask 'Have we met before?' or 'Have I not seen you before?' Often we establish links of commonality between ourselves and others during set induction and during continuing conversation: 'Oh! I'm a nurse too'; 'We live in the same street then'; 'Do you work at Snodgrass Incorporated as well.' Various phrases such as 'breaking the ice', 'chatting up' or 'making contact' indicate this set-induction behaviour. The amorous male's comment 'Haven't I seen you somewhere before?', has been so commonly used it is now a redundant cliché. Even comments such as 'Have you got a light?' and 'Have you got the time?' can be treated with some suspicion, because of their set-inducing potential.

Providing 'creature comforts'

Offering a drink, a comfortable chair, confectionery or the like can assist set induction. Nurses often offer to rearrange pillows or offer a drink when approaching a patient. Indeed, any helping activity may induce conversation if the opportunity is taken. It is possible for the nurse to carry out many helping activities without engaging in real conversation. It is common for nurses to restrict utterances to instructions and meaningless comment, rather than use the oppor-tunity to enter into a conversation.

The second area of conversational skill involves maintaining conversational interaction. This will be achieved by securing and maintaining rapport, an understanding of turn-taking behaviour and an avoidance of errors that may spoil the conversational process.

Maintaining Conversation – Rapport

Achieving and maintaining rapport is in itself a nursing social skill. The over-used statements 'Achieve rapport with the patient' or 'Form a relationship with a patient' seem to prevent us asking two questions, 'What is it?' and 'How do we do it?'. Rapport is concerned with mutual recognition of each other's interactional needs, acknowledging them, communicating to the other person that you realize his or her needs and meeting them wherever possible.

Take, for instance, a situation in which a patient has a need to relieve emotional tension by talking and the nurse does not allow this, by dominating the discussion with a one-sided drawn-out monologue. The basic requirements for rapport have not been met. The nurse did not recognize the patient's need. The patient soon realizes this, becomes frustrated, discontinues the interaction and holds a recollection of a dissatisfying encounter. This dissatisfaction is seen as one of the characteristics of the nurse as a person and the patient is less likely to enter into social contact with that nurse again. So rapport involves checking the feeling state of the other, by observing vocal and body signals. It involves letting the other person know you understand his or her feelings about the encounter.

Finally, one needs to alter one's own behaviour to satisfy the other person's needs in the interaction. Needless to say, there is a two-way process in every one-to-one human interaction.

Maintaining Conversation – Turn-taking

Conversation involves a 'give and take' convention. This is such a fundamental process that it has been identified as a skill that predisposes in infancy to vocal language production (see Silverstein, in Bruner, 1974). During the prelinguistic stage, interactions are conversational in nature even before the child is able to speak (Snow, 1977). Language ability is, in fact, developed from an ability to take turns in conversation.

A mother's speech and interaction with her baby demonstrate early turn-taking behaviour. Mothers speak short sentences and stop as if to allow the infant a conversational turn. The 3-month-old infant cannot speak but appears to become more active, increasing facial expression, gurgling and making distinctive mouth movements that look like attempts to speak. A mother has a tendency to interpret these and often takes the infant's turn for him, providing answers to her own questions or asking herself questions. This would be considered strange speech behaviour in any other context (Snow, 1977).

Sacks *et al.* (1974) describe two components of turn-taking in conversation. The turn-constructional component is determined by the construction of speech. The end of a sentence is an example of an appropriate place for a person to take his turn. Turn-allocation is achieved when a new speaker begins to speak or the present speaker takes another 'turn'. Self-selection is achieved by speaking first. Various utterances by their very nature suggest to the other person that he should take his turn. Forms of turn-allocation response include questions, compliments, insults and greetings.

Argyle (1972) has found that looking is an important cue during conversations. During conversation two people achieve eye contact on several occasions. Each person's direction of gaze can meet so that they look at each other's eyes and faces simultaneously. Sometimes, looking is one-sided, for instance when the other person looks away. People tend to look about twice as much while they are listening as when they are talking. Looking shows another person that one is interested in him. Exline and Winters (1965) discovered that people look more at people that they like. Argyle (1972) states that shifts of gaze regulate the synchronization of speech.

It is important to remember the power of eye contact for maintaining conversation. Looking at the other person's face tends to occur in the speaker just as he or she begins. At the end of sentences or phrases he or she looks up briefly, while at the end of a long utterance he or she tends to prolong his gaze (Argyle, 1972). Kendon (1967) found that looking is an important mechanism for stopping input from the listener while formulating another sentence. It is a mechanism for controlling the listener's behaviour. It signals the speaker's intention to hold the floor. If he prolongs his gaze towards the listener at the end of utterances he is signalling his willingness to allow the other to speak. The listener can also indicate frustration by looking away. This then becomes a request to the other person to stop speaking so that the listener may begin to speak. While eye contact and looking may be a sign of heightened interest, too much of it may be unpleasant and embarrassing (Argyle, 1972). One should, therefore, never overuse looking as intentional behaviour during conversation, even though it is an important skill for maintaining conversation.

Maintaining Conversation – Non-verbal Cues

Other non-verbal cues help to maintain conversation. Facing in the direction of the other, close proximity, facial expression, head-nodding and gestures all serve to signal to the other person that one is willing to maintain the interaction. Vocal/verbal cues such as 'Mmm', 'Uhuh',

'Go on' and 'That's interesting' help to maintain conversation, as do questions and other exclamations. The content of the conversation also has important motivational properties. We are all familiar with a reluctance to communicate because we are not interested or cannot understand what the other person is saying.

Errors in Communication

The errors described below are modified and extended from Weinhold and Elliott (1979); they have important implications for maintaining conversation.

1. Generalization errors:
   (a) Saying 'one' or 'people' or 'you'.
   (b) Using words like 'always' or 'never' to support a point of view.
   (c) Picking one example as proof of a general phenomenon: 'Nobody teaches nurses in this hospital, Sister Sproggins didn't.'
2. Confusions:
   (a) Confusing inference and observation (fact).
   (b) Confusing feedback with confrontation.
   (c) Confusing judgemental behaviour with feedback behaviour. Making judgements instead of giving feedback.
   (d) Confusing feelings with thoughts (saying 'I feel' to mean 'I think').
3. Indirectness:
   (a) Asking a question instead of making a statement.
   (b) Making a statement instead of asking, e.g. 'I wish I could have a drink of water'.
   (c) Saying 'have to' and 'should' to mean 'choose to' or 'want to'.
   (d) Answering a question with another question.
   (e) Saying 'I guess' and 'Maybe' when you are certain.
   (f) Saying 'try' instead of 'do'.
4. Frustrating the other person:
   (a) Talking about a person and not to him or her (e.g. to a mother, ignoring the child, to an aide rather than to the blind person, to the relative rather than the patient).
   (b) Interrupting the speaker.
   (c) Changing the subject.
   (d) Chaining. Listening to just enough of what others say, then changing to a topic that interests oneself.
   (e) Talking too much.
   (f) Not sharing. Keeping the focus on oneself rather than on others, e.g. talking about one's own experiences and problems, to the exclusion of the other person's concerns.

(g) Being directive and preventing personal equality.

5. Personal defence strategy:
   (a) Blaming one's own feelings on someone else.
   (b) Discounting some aspect of a situation.
   (c) Maintaining a position of passivity instead of actively taking responsibility for oneself and one's own behaviour.

6. Unhelpful orientation:
   (a) Rescuing by doing something for someone that he or she can do for himself or herself.
   (b) Entering into interpersonal competition in which a win-or-lose outcome or one-upmanship is inevitable.

Set Closure

To complete conversational skill, nurses should learn to discontinue conversations leaving patients relatively safe and content, having satisfied their needs and at an appropriate moment. Several ways for ending conversations can be employed. Hargie *et al.* (1981) suggest the following set closures appropriate to conversational skill:

1. Non-task related statements. These statements change the topic of conversation to something fairly superficial. Statements such as 'Well, at least it's a nice day outside', 'See you tomorrow' and 'I hope everything turns out OK', take the focus of attention away from the topic of conversation.
2. Social acknowledgement statements. Comments such as 'Well, it's been nice talking to you', 'I hope we meet again' and 'Thank you for talking to me' acknowledge the importance of the other person while marking an end to the conversation.
3. Motivating statements. Examples include 'Well, see what you can do', 'It's up to you to make your mind up' and 'We'll try that and see where we go from there'. These statements incite action and indicate that there is little point in carrying on the conversation until this action is taken.
4. Verbal closure markers, such as 'Goodbye', 'Cheerio', 'Bye-bye', 'Cheers', 'See you' and 'All the best!'. Some are more direct, such as 'You can go now', 'I'll have to go now' and 'I can't sit talking all day'.
5. Non-verbal closure markers. These include changes in body posture, orientation or proximity. We have discussed the effect of looking away earlier and it may be used to close a conversation. Standing up, fidgeting, clock-watching and moving towards the door are also obvious changes in behaviour that cause set closure. Some behaviours such as hand-shaking and waving are more direct.

WRITING SKILLS

Writing is the permanent representation of language using specially contrived characters that symbolize so far as possible the original speech form. The written language form differs from the spoken form in several ways. Writing is permanent and does not fade as do spoken cues. It is permanent, i.e. until the recording material is destroyed (e.g. paper by fire).   The exact message may be read over and over again. Speech messages are never heard again in exactly the same form, even if repeated. Speech messages may now be recorded but reproduction of the original sounds is rarely exact.

Since writing is permanent, the rate of message reception is controlled by the receiver, whereas the rate of reception in speech is largely dictated by the speaker. We can read slowly or quickly, but we can only pick up the spoken message as slowly or as quickly as the person is speaking. Speech is most often perceived in the presence of the speaker and writing is most frequently not. There are some exceptions to both these points – for instance, tape-recorded message, telephone conversation, and somebody giving a person a letter or essay that has been written to be read in the author's presence. These situations are uncommon and with telephone speech both parties interact, albeit at a distance. It is still most often the case that the recipient of the spoken message can ask for immediate clarification, whereas the recipient of the written message cannot ask the author for immediate clarification. Written messages are also de-contextualized; they cannot add to the communication efficiency by using environmental references because writer and reader are not sharing the same environment. Because of this, writing must be more elaborate and explicit.

It can be suggested that Bernstein's elaborated code is effective for written communication, whereas restricted code is highly ineffective. The following message is meaningless because it is context-dependent: 'What is this, what is it doing here?', 'It could be ours '. The reader cannot specify the object of the discussion or who the possible owners are. The reader may add information from other contextual sources – e.g. experience, knowledge or imagination – to make sense of the statement. It is not uncommon for this sort of addition to take place when written messages are difficult to understand.

Writing, because of its permanence, can pass information from one generation to another. The dead person's will and testament can make wishes known after his or her death. Events in the past (e.g. industrial events, revolution, the Battle of Hastings, the Boston Tea Party) can be shared by readers hundreds of years later. Written messages lack the non-verbal and 'paralinguistic' features of speech and thus lose some of the communicative sophistication of speech. Another feature of writing is it cumulative nature. A nursing student's lecture notes are a case in point. If he or she does not take notes from spoken lectures most of the information is lost. When notes are taken, information accumulates and he or she can add to it or elaborate information already recorded.

Writing Skills in Nursing

There are several situations in which writing skill becomes crucial in nursing practice. The list below will serve to outline the most common situations in which skilled written communication is necessary:

- nursing care plan;
- nursing care reports, including evaluative reports;
- writing letters for disabled patients;
- accident reports or reports of untoward incidents;
- applications for equipment, building modifications or extra staff;
- person descriptions in cases of missing or absent patients.
- letters to fellow professionals;
- essays for studentship and examination purposes;
- papers for publication.

Guidelines for Writing Skills

Nurses should bear in mind that they are always communicating with at least one person and sometimes many people when using writing skill. When the other person is not physically present, we sometimes forget that the object of our communication is another person. Since writing is de-contextualized it must be explicit and explanation should be carried out conscientiously . The responsibility is with the writer to assess how it will be interpreted by the reader. There is also some compulsion to be precise and factual. As written messages are permanent they may be reproduced long after the thoughts and intentions of the writer have passed by. The writer can be held accountable and responsible for the things he or she has written for many years after carrying out this communicative act. The following guidelines may serve to assist the nurse who wishes to develop writing skill.

Predict the likely readership

This is important because one may choose inappropriate terminology or phrase structure, making understanding difficult for those who need to use the written message. Sometimes attitudes and special knowledge (context) may not be shared by the author and readers. A nurse may have particular problems in justifying expenditure in writing to the finance officer, when he or she does not share nursing values, experiences or patterns of thinking. This principle is also appropriate to nursing records (which may be read by junior nurse), applications, letters, or papers for publication.

Plan the layout

With short statements, this may simply mean considering phrase structure, accurate spelling and word selection. This means thinking before writing. Flesch (1964) suggests that sentences of about 11 words are easily read, while sentences of over 25 words are difficult to understand. Larger written messages such as letters, formal reports, papers for publication and examination essays require the author to give some organized structure to the account to facilitate reading and understanding for the recipient.

A simple way of organizing a long written account is to begin by drawing up a simple plan. This can involve making a 'shopping list' of points to be made. Each entry should be just one or two words long to allow the writer to recall the main discussion areas.

When answering an examination question, one may produce an essay plan for nursing care of the unconscious patient by generating the following list (not, in this example, intended to be complete):

Position
Safety
Eye pads
Pupil reactions
Intravenous therapy
Level of consciousness
Hygiene
Excretion

These points may be rearranged and numbered so that some sensible order is produced:

1. Position
   (a) Safety.
   (b) Eye pads.
2. Intravenous therapy.
3. Hygiene.
4. Excretion.
5. Pupil reactions.
6. Level of consciousness.

Each point can now be taken in numerical order.

More extended technical accounts, such as open essays, reports and journal articles may be organized under three basic headings:

1. Introduction – setting the scene, reasons, background.
2. Main body – main points to be made.
3. Conclusion – finishing by drawing points together, commenting on relationships to other work etc.

When written accounts become extremely long, other sections may be added to help the reader assess which part he wants to pay most attention to, which part he wants to omit or even whether he wants to read the paper at all. Such additions may give headings such as:

1. List of contents.
2. Brief summary of whole paper.
3. Introduction.
4. Main body.
5. Conclusions.

If published work has been mentioned, a list of references should be included at the end. References are usually listed in alphabetical order of author's surname. For each reference the surname is entered, followed by initials, year of publication in brackets, title or paper, journal name and issue, publishers (for books) and page number (if crucial). Examples can be found in the list of references at the end of this book.

If material would cause distraction or confusion in the main body of the account, one can place it at the end of the whole paper as an appendix. The appendix number would then be referred to in the main body of the paper. Management and government reports often do this.

Legibility

Words, letters and symbols should be written clearly. This involves learning and practice, initially to develop the person's handwriting style. If personal script handwriting is poor, one should print. Really crucial communications should be typed. Ballpoint pens encourage lax style and using a fountain pen may encourage the writer to take more care because of the wet ink and broad nib. Most handwriting can be improved by taking time and care. Writing should not be so small that reading causes strain for the reader.

Relevance

The information in a written communication should be relevant at two levels. The first level involves the total content. The content should fit the aims of the written message. If an examination question asks the examinee to discuss the preoperative care of a particular condition, there is little point writing about the postoperative care or the surgical technique that will be adopted. Similarly, nursing records should be an account of the process of nursing, not an additional medical (doctor's) record. At the second level, relevance should be maintained by avoiding any tendency to stray from the point. One should avoid such diversion that will necessitate a radical return to earlier discussion and a resulting break in train of thought.

Continuity

This principle is related to points made about planning and relevance. Any long written account should have an unbroken thread of logically related points from beginning to end. The reader should understand the relationship between the point being made, the previous discussion and the forthcoming discussion. An unbroken thread of continuity can be maintained by using communication markers or signposts that tell the reader how the forthcoming point is related to the previous point. This takes the form of an explanation to the reader of what you are about to discuss, giving a reason and a link with previous discussion. An example will help to demonstrate this point. Imagine that a paper has described the need for problem-solving ability in nursing and the author thinks it appropriate to point out the complexity of studying problem-solving ability. He or she may begin his next paragraph in this way: 'A cognitive study carried out by Wason (1968) consisted of a four-card problem, in which he asked respondents to . . .'.

The reader is likely to wonder why the author has suddenly started talking about psychological experimentation and why he suddenly mentions Wason and this four-card problem. The following sentence may ease the reader into the next point and give direction to the discussion: 'Now that the need for problem-solving ability in nursing has been defined, it is useful to examine the complexity of the concept of problem-solving before discussing the characteristics of problem-solving skill. An experiment by Wason (1968) demonstrates the complex nature of problem-solving skill.'

This is, in fact, a link statement and a justification of the change in thought. If the thread of continuity is broken too many times the reader may become disinterested or confused.

Accuracy

Written messages must be factual and precise. Rough estimation and vague terminology not only cause problems for the reader who needs to use the account, but also for the author if she is to be held responsible for the content at a later date. If a person has injured himself at 10.30 a.m., one should write this down, not a broad statement such as 'earlier this morning' or 'at coffee time'. Nurses should not guess facts when they are unsure. Sometimes the need for accuracy requires checking and considerable effort. This may involve questioning other people, looking up words in a dictionary or a literature search. The habit of maintaining accuracy is a worthwhile pursuit in the long term.

A different perspective on accuracy is concerned with the communication of fact, inference or value judgement. Wherever possible, one should indicate clearly when content has been inferred from the facts by the author. Inference goes beyond the facts to make interpretations or guesses. This information will be influenced by the author's judgement and is likely to be subjective rather than objective. A nurse, in writing a report of an incident on the ward, may write: 'John jumped up and walked over to the nurse as if to do her harm'. The last part of the phrase is an inference and may be unjustly pointing to violent tendencies in John when, in actual fact, he means none.

If inferences are to be included in written nursing accounts, one should make them on the basis of informed opinion and it should be pointed out in the text that the author's opinion has been expressed. Phrases such as 'I thought that', 'in my opinion' and 'it seemed to me that', will help to mark out inference statements.

Facts, wherever possible, should be substantiated by confirmation from other sources. If two people agree on an observation, they should be mentioned in the account. If a fact is based on expert opinion or research findings, reference should be made to the appropriate source. Finally, personal value judgements of the author should be considered carefully before being included in any document that is likely to influence others. An author's values are usually easily identified. They are personal estimations of worth, of right or wrong, good or bad, acceptability or unacceptability, of any particular issue. It is because values vary so much from one individual to another and are mainly associated with the individual characteristics of the person expressing them that they are frequently worth less in any objective written account. An expression of personal values should be carried out only after assessing the function that will be served by this personal expression. This can also be marked out as a personal value in the paper in an obvious way.

Terminology

One should use words or terms that the reader can understand. Whenever possible the most common word should be chosen when several alternatives are available. Technical terms must be used when scientific or semantic precision is required. They should not be used to

~~nress,~~ confuse or place the reader at any personal disadvantage. ⎢⎢⎢ this is the use of abbreviations; these are open to ⎢⎢⎢ ~~etation~~ and should be avoided wherever possible.

Always communicate

⎢⎢ n strange to suggest that one can write a message without ⎢⎢ ~~ting.~~ Examples of this, however, are often found when ⎢⎢ ssages become routine. If a nursing record says 'no change' ⎢⎢ every entry, page after page, who knows what the original state of the person was? It is inconceivable that change has not occurred in any aspect of the patient's life. Such messages communicate lack of knowledge or lack of interest. They may prevent others reading them because they induce an expectation of uselessness. One should always write something meaningful, not write for the sake of writing, or to satisfy some routine.

THE SKILL OF TOUCHING

Touch is one of the five senses and it helps us to gather much information throughout life. It has been mentioned briefly above in the discussion of non-verbal communication. Touch is a particularly important means of communication for children. it is important for development in the early stages of life, both in developing tactile sensory ability and in gathering information about the outside world (Frank, 1957). Harlow (1971) discovered the harmful effects of depriving infant monkeys of touch sensation in infancy. They became non-social and were unable to perform the sex act in later life. Other work tends to suggest harmful effects in human children (Chapin, 1915; Talbot, 1941; Montague, 1971). Some have suggested possible fatal consequences of touch deprivation in children (Montague, 1971).

Touching tends to decrease as children become older, particularly in Western societies (Jourard, 1966). This results in the reluctance of many adults to engage in touching behaviour because it comes to have either sexual or invasive connotations. Touch tends to increase in adolescence as sexual interest becomes more significant, and its sexual connotations are probably the greatest obstacle to the beneficial use of touch in our society. Touching others tends to communicate the following things:

- sexual interest;
- friendliness;
- intimacy and familiarity;
- nature of the relationship;

- occupation of toucher;
- social conventions;
- aggression;
- concern;
- affection.

Nurses work in an occupation where touch is of major importance and they are given permission by society to engage in more intimate touching behaviour in pursuit of this occupation (Figure 3.6). Passing suppositories and catheterisation are examples of extremely intimate touching behaviours. The nurse is only granted this permission in certain situations and set induction is an important skill that sets the scene for these situations. Explanation by the nurse is important to justify touching patients. Mason and Pratt (1980) and Pratt and Mason (1981) have suggested that nurses may help patients accept various deformities and unsightly abnormalities by touching or handling the part that causes consternation. In this way they can minimize the patient's feelings of being unacceptable or incomplete. Acceptable touching is an important means of reassuring the patient and this mode of reassuring is often sadly lacking in everyday practice. Mason and Pratt (1980) also suggest that touch helps some patients to maintain contact with their physical world: 'When the patient is semiconscious, withdrawn or perhaps unable to communicate or understand others, the medium of touch is a natural and powerful means of bringing him into the 'here and now'.

The occasions when nurses use touch can be summarized by the following list:

- to move the patient or parts of his or her body;
- to support the patient physically;
- to carry out practical procedures on the patient;
- to carry out observations (e.g. pulse);
- to reassure the patient;
- to keep the patient in contact with his or her world;
- to communicate attitudes and intentions;
- to communicate with infants and older children;
- to restrain violent or self-destructive patients.

As a social skill, the nurse's touching style is learned and not inherited. When learning touching style in nursing, the nurse acquires it from three separate sources: (i) the nurse's cultural background; (ii) the nursing school; and (iii) the nurse–patient interaction (Estabrookes and Morse, 1992).

When carrying out intimate touching behaviour, whether it be cuddling a child, lifting a patient or passing a suppository, several principles may be followed:

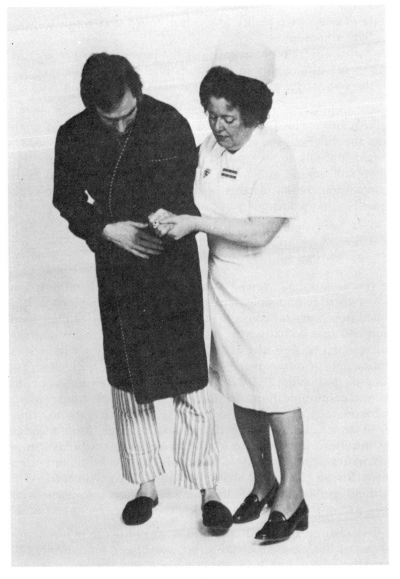

Figure 3.6 Nursing involves touching.

1. Identify the need for touching. This ensures mainly that the nurses keep in mind what they are doing and why they are doing it.
2. Explain to the patient what is to happen and why.
3. Ask the patient's permission to touch.
4. Observe social and cultural conventions. Do not cause embarrassment or misunderstanding by choosing inappropriate touching behaviour.
5. Apologize for touching accidents. This involves inappropriate or embarrassing touching incidents.
6. Be aware of one's own ability to use firm touch and gentle touch in appropriate situations.
7. Ensure privacy and do not overexpose the patient. These things add to feelings of vulnerability in situations of touch.
8. Thank the patient for allowing this intimacy.

Estabrookes and Morse (1992) further describe three steps in the touching sequence. The first is the talking stage, the second is the talking and the touching stage, and the third is the touching stage. The nurse should just talk to the patient first, e.g. give explanation, then touch while still talking and finally the patient may accept touching without verbal interaction. At this point, the communicative power of touching will be at its greatest.

INTRAPERSONAL COMMUNICATION

Previous discussion has viewed communication as something that goes on between two people, an interpersonal phenomenon. It is worthwhile, however, to consider another fact about human communication and that is that we are all able to receive information from and about ourselves. We can actually communicate with ourselves. The phenomenon of intrapersonal communication has been described by Weinhold and Elliott (1979) as an essential requirement for interpersonal communication. In their discussion of transpersonal communication they describe self-awareness as the 'degree to which you are in touch with yourself, your body, and your feelings, thoughts, intuitions and behaviour'. In the subsequent discussion on social skill in this book, self-awareness will emerge as an important requirement for all the social skills. Nurses will constantly need to monitor their personal functioning and reactions. Awareness of themselves will enable nurses to do three things:

1. Make decisions on the most appropriate responses to make.
2. Assess his or her personal abilities but, even more importantly, the inadequacies that would be reduced by personal development and training.

3. Obtain feedback on personal performance during skilled action.

Weinhold and Elliott (1979) identified the following intrapersonal processes:

- awareness of internal sensations, including body awareness breathing and tension;
- awareness of feelings;
- awareness of thoughts;
- awareness of wants and needs;
- here-and-now awareness;
- awareness of past influences;
- awareness of unfinished business;
- awareness of dreams and fantasies;
- intuitive processes;
- intrapersonal problem-solving.

It may be obvious that this concept of self-awareness is also relevant to Chapter 2 on assessing the person. Indeed, self-awareness is the result of personal assessment. How then can one assess oneself? There are two major sources of information on the self, interoception and introspection.

Interoception

Interoceptors are sensory nerve endings that are located in the tissues of the body. They provide information about internal activity. There are three types of interoceptor: (i) visceroceptors, which provide information about the internal organs; (ii) chemoreceptors (e.g. carotid and aortic bodies), which provide information about chemical changes in the body; and (iii) proprioceptors, which supply information about the tension of muscles and tendons in the locomotor system. Most of the interoceptive information coming from our body is not, however, available to our awareness. The information that we are aware of is concerned mainly with pain and tension (stretch receptors). Some activities that can help us to appreciate more of our internal sensations are listed at the end of this chapter. Common body sensations that we can all become aware of are breathing, heartbeat, pulsation of arteries, muscle fatigue, distension of the stomach, rectum and bladder and sensations associated with emotions, such as 'butterflies in the stomach' and tremor in anxiety.

Introspection

Introspection is the act of exploring one's own conscious mental experiences. There are many things available to conscious awareness – thoughts, emotions, memories, images (pictures in the mind), attitudes, needs, problems, wishes and problem-solving processes. One problem associated with introspection should always be borne in mind, however. This is that much mental activity is unconscious. This fact was perhaps Freud's most significant discovery (Freud, 1940). He described 'unconscious mental activity', as that completely inaccessible to our awareness and 'preconscious mental activity', ideas which are unconscious but can be recalled with some effort. It is perhaps worthwhile to say that an understanding about the existence of unconscious mental activity is in itself an aid to self-awareness. In this way, the person can acknowledge that he or she may have thoughts and motives of which he or she is totally unaware. While Freud's theory is still highly controversial, it is still worthwhile examining his work so that one can get some idea of the possible content and effect of unconscious mental activity. Once again activities described at the end of this chapter will help in the understanding of self-awareness by introspection.

A final point about self-awareness is that when one begins to look closely at oneself it is likely that several inadequacies and deficiencies will become apparent. It is very easy to ignore them and find excuses, so it may be necessary to learn how to accept and cope with these deficiencies. This may be achieved by extra knowledge, understanding and even counselling from someone expert in helping people to accept personal feedback.

REFLECTIVE ACTIVITIES

1. During a television play in which there are two people in conversation turn the sound down and for a 2-min period note all the transmission channels you can observe. For an additional 2-min period turn down the brightness so that the picture is obliterated but the sound is on. This time note the characteristics of the speech.
2. When people come to you and ask you questions at work, try to decide what communicative function they are trying to achieve, provided that you have time to reflect. Keep a checklist of functions in your pocket.
3. Next time you leave a message, no matter how trivial, for someone, see if you can satisfy the eight criteria for sending messages efficiently.
4. When answering the telephone see if you can use the four principles for receiving messages effectively.
5. Whenever you notice a situation in which there is a mistake or misunderstanding in communication, or when you have had difficulty communicating with someone else, decide which type of

communication failure has occurred. Also decide what remedial action was taken or could be taken.

6. Next time you are tempted to begin a conversation, stop for a moment and ask yourself how you are starting the conversation. How has this encounter with the other person been entered into? Try a method of set induction that you do not normally use.

7. During a conversation see if you can note:
   (a) Non-verbal signals that maintain the conversation.
   (b) Turn-taking behaviour.
   (c) Patterns of eye contact at the beginning and end of sentences both when listening and talking.

8. Using a taped conversation between two people (with their permission or from impromptu television/radio dialogue), try to identify communication errors described in the section on conversation.

9. Notice how you or others break off conversations. This will be much easier in those situations where it is obvious that one person is eager to get away.

10. Try to write a paper for the nursing press, perhaps a care study or case history. Use the guidelines for writing skill. See if you can get it published in the popular nursing press. (Do not be disappointed if it is rejected – first attempts often are.)

11. During a span of duty note each time you touch a patient and note where you touched him or her and why.

12. Lay on your back on the floor with your hands by your side.
    (a) See if you can become aware of your heart beating.
    (b) Take a deep breath inward until you cannot breathe in any more. Feel the tension in the lungs – you may even experience a slight pain.
    (c) Tense all the muscles in your body. While you do this concentrate on the feeling in the various muscles.
    (d) After tensing all the muscles in your body relax as completely as possible. Concentrate on the feeling as you relax and during the relaxed state.
    (e) Close your eyes and stretch your arms out on either side of you with the back of your hands touching the floor. Point the first finger of each hand and slowly bring the fingers of each hand together in front of you. Keep your arms stretched out in front of you. Do this very slowly and concentrate on the feeling in each of the muscles in your hands and arms. Did your fingers meet?

13. After reading the previous task, did you do it, consider doing it and pass on to this activity or did you say that you do not intend doing that sort of thing?
    (a) If you did the task ask yourself how you felt while doing it –

excited, silly, interested, self-conscious or what? Did you do the task on your own or with friends? Why?

(b) If you do not intend to carry out the task consider your reasons for this reluctance.

14. Next time you become anxious, sit back for a moment, close your eyes and concentrate on the sensations in your body. What are you thinking about as you worry? Perhaps you could repeat this for other emotions such as anger, excitement, jealousy, happiness and misery.

15. When you next go to bed, wait until you are fully relaxed then let your mind wander. Stop every now and then to consider your thoughts. If you dream during the night try to remember the content of your dreams the next day. See if you can tell yourself in a dream that you must remember a particular thing; some people can do this.

16. Sit down and make a list of your strengths and weaknesses, the goods things about you and the bad. Put the attributes on one side of the sheet and the faults on the other. Try to make sure that your lists are long and contain an equal number of items – i.e. your faults' list should be as long as your strengths' list. If you are really brave, show your list to other people and see if they agree.

17. Make up another list but this time write down all your hopes for the future and disappointments from the past.

18. Think of a person whom you dislike intensely. Ask yourself what it is about **you** that causes you to dislike him. What are you prepared to do and what are you not prepared to do to improve your relationship? Why are you reluctant to do some of the things you have thought of?

19. Write down what you think of yourself. Are you good-looking, intelligent, witty, happy-go-lucky, sociable, friendly, considerate, sexy, emotionally stable and secure. Or are you just honest.

SELF-EVALUATION TASKS

Do not read any of these questions until you are sure that you understand the material in the previous section.

1. Draw a diagram to show a human communication model.
2. List eight functions for nurse–patient communication.
3. List and briefly describe four principles for receiving a message efficiently.
4. List principles for rectifying communication failures.
5. Briefly describe five methods of set closure applicable to conversation.

6. List and describe eight principles for touching behaviour in nursing practice.
7. List the types of information that may be obtained in intrapersonal communication.

Check on your answers in the text.

CHAPTER 4

Self-reflection

LEARNING OBJECTIVES

You should concentrate on being able to:

1. Acquire a positive attitude to yourself.
2. Describe the humanist approach to self-reflection.
3. Analyse the different ways in which you and other people describe themselves.
4. Differentiate between the public self, private self, self-concept, actual self and ideal self.
5. Seek feedback from other people, self-reflection exercises and psychometric tests with a positive attitude to your personal development.
6. Accept the existence of the hidden aspects of the self and constraints on total self-awareness, from a psychoanalytical viewpoint.
7. Be aware of the part that the concepts of mental defence mechanism and dream analysis could play in self-reflection.
8. Describe the contribution that skills of self-reflection can make to nursing practise.

WHAT IS SELF-REFLECTION?

The process of self-reflection is included in this account of social skills, not because it deals with an analysis of interpersonal transactions but because it is an important requisite sub-skill for the successful practice of nursing social skills. The end of the previous chapter on communication proposed that we can communicate with ourselves. This chapter carries on this theme by developing the general contention that the nurse can become more aware of his or her self and of the helpful and unhelpful facets of his or her consistent self presentation to others.

Before the reader begins to anticipate any problems associated with some uncompromising discovery of the self, it is worth suggesting a few attitudinal ground rules in an effort to avoid any downward spirals of self-recrimination that occur all too often in our reflections about ourselves. It is advisable to remember that all human beings are unique and that we are unique because we are each made up of an enormous number of attributes. Each of our attributes may have positive or negative affects on other people.

The quiet person who is not outspoken may not make contributions in group work situations but may be valued by their friends and acquaintances for their ability to listen. In a similar way we can view our personal qualities as being of potential use in some situations in life and of being a hindrance in others. Often we use the phrase 'personal strengths and weaknesses'.

One should remember that no human being can ever be infallible and self recrimination can never change this aspect of human nature. In fact if we were all perfect we would be insipid and the nature of our humanity would be lost. We would all be like robots. It is because of our imperfections that being human can be so exciting. It can be argued that the aim of self-reflection is to maximize the positive effects we have on ourselves and others as well as minimizing the negative effects. We do not aim to replace ourselves with a better person, we aim to maximize our own human potential. These sentiments are aptly described in some of the of the writing of Max Ehrmann (1983) in his philosophical statement, the *'Desiderata'* and also Rudyard Kipling in his famous poem entitled *'If'*.

> If you compare yourself with others,
> you may become vain and bitter; for
> always there will be greater and
> lesser persons than yourself.
>
> Enjoy your achievements as well
> as your plans.
>
> Be yourself. Especially do not feign
> affection.
>
> Nurture strength of spirit to shield
> you in sudden misfortune.
> But do not distress yourself with
> imaginings. Many fears are born of
> fatigue and loneliness.
>
> Beyond a wholesome discipline be
> gentle with yourself.
>
> *Ehrmann, 1983*

If you can dream – and not make dreams your master,
If you can think – and not make thoughts your aim,
If you can meet with Triumph and Disaster,
And treat those two impostors just the same. . .

If you can talk with crowds and keep your virtue,
Or walk with Kings – nor lose the common touch,
If neither foes nor loving friends can hurt you,
If all men count with you, but none too much;
If you can fill the unforgiving minute
With sixty seconds' worth of distance run,
Yours is the Earth and everything that's in it. . .
Rudyard Kipling, 1910

Feeling good about yourself is not a luxury; it is an absolute necessity.
Palladino, 1989

The process of self-reflection should be positive (Figure 4.1) and we should constantly consider how to maximize our attributes and positive potential. The discussion that follows will try to equip nurses with a vocabulary so that they have a greater capacity to talk about themselves, there will be some ideas that facilitate self-understanding and some methods that will assist the nurse to make decisions about his or her 'self' and the contribution that his or her 'self' can make towards helping other people. At certain times the text will recommend that the reader attempt the activities listed at the end of this chapter. The purpose of this is to provide some objective stimulus for self-reflection. Some of these activities will not provide accurate feedback if the reader continues to read the text rather than do the activity first. If an understanding of the interpretation of the activity is acquired first the reader may find her/himself finding out what she/he would like to be rather than gaining a more accurate insight into the self.

WHO ARE YOU?

Yes a very strange question but one that has been asked by many psychologists and one in particular will help to clarify why this question is useful to the nurse for self-reflection (Zurcher, 1977). The approach that begins this discussion derives from humanist psychology (Rogers, 1951). The humanist approach says that you are who you say you are. The understanding of a person's humanity resides within the person themselves. No other human being can know more about oneself than oneself. Before this discussion continues the reader is asked to complete Activity 1 at the end of this chapter. Given that the activity has been completed it is now possible to emphasize that this method of self-reflection is useful not just because people list specific facts that they see as most important (and that no two people produce identical lists of facts) but that people also describe themselves in different ways and this also says much about the person.

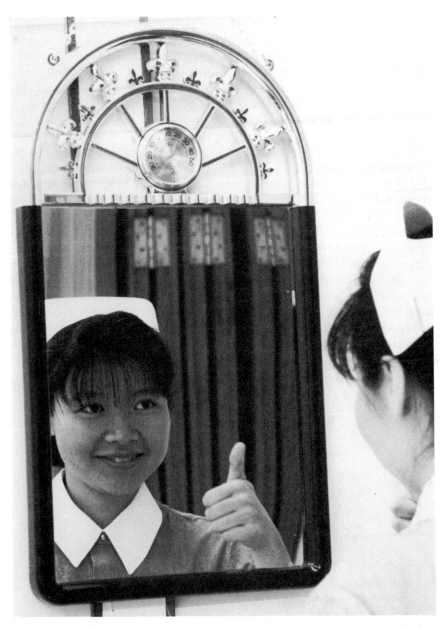

Figure 4.1 Feeling good about yourself is not a luxury, it is an absolute necessity.

Zurcher found that there were four types of description people gave when they undertook the *'Twenty Statements'* problem (McPartland, 1965). These types of description combine in various ways and at different times to form the mutable self. The self that changes and the self that is adaptable. The forms of description are: (i) the physical self; (ii) the social self; (iii) the reflective self; and (iv) the oceanic self. The **physical self**, which can be detected in descriptions that refer to body sensations, image and biographical details. The statements "I am 6 feet tall', "I live in a small village' provide good examples of this category of description. Items on the list that describe roles or relationships with other people are presenting the *social self*. These descriptions are socially defined and can be socially validated. "I am a mother', "I am a nurse', "I am middle class' all represent the social self. The **reflective self** is demonstrated in items that are situation free, they do not describe specific behaviours but styles of behaviour. "I am a thoughtful person' or "I dislike pushy people' indicate the reflective self.

The **oceanic self** includes all those descriptions of oneself that are to some extent fanciful and vague – they are statements that are so comprehensive that they do not enable others to understand any particular feature of the person. A statement such as 'I am a pebble on the beach of time' (Figure 4.2) indicates the sort of descriptions described as oceanic self. After doing the *'Twenty Statements'* problem the reader will find that a the list that they have produced may provide more items under some categories and none under others. If this exercise is repeated after a year or two the reader will notice some

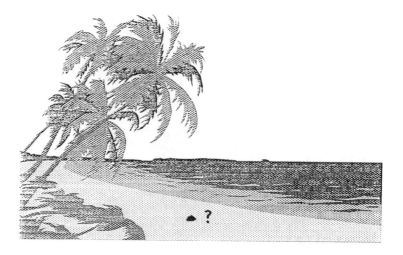

Figure 4.2 Who am I?

changes. It is even more interesting to ask your friends or fellow students to do the *'Twenty Statements'* problem and to compare their lists with your own. It is not interesting because we find out more about other people but because we begin to understand more about how different we are to other people. This is where we have one basis for self-reflection.

Before proceeding go to the end of this chapter and do Activity 2.

WHO DO I THINK I AM?

The lists that have been generated in Activity 2 will help us to understand some important variables in self concept that have been called 'two motives and four selves' (Baumeister and Tice, 1986). Many scholars of the self agree that our self-image behaviour is directed towards, on the one hand, the presentation of ourselves to an audience (other people) and on the other to the construction of the sort of person we think we should be. Many nurses will recognize that when they are nursing they are different to their usual selves. When they are playing to the audiences (patients and colleagues) their real self may be modified. If the reader also recognizes this then he or she has some experience of the two processes that influence our self-reflection.

These motives give rise to conceptions about four types of self (Baumeister and Tice, 1986). There is the public self and the private self. The private self can further be subdivided into the self-concept, the actual self and the ideal self. The **public self** is that which is known to others. It is often conveyed in the idea of personal reputation. Indeed the public self is open to observation by anyone.

The **private self**, however, is the opposite, it is that which is not open to observation by others. More specifically it entails the ability (or the right) to control who can view one's own behaviour (Tedeschi, 1986). It is said to have three meanings. The first is the **self-concept**. This is said to be somewhat secretive and there is an automatic assumption that others see us in a different way to the way we see ourselves. This is why Activity 2 asks you to list all the ways other people would describe yourself. There is also an assumption associated with the idea of self-concept that the person can deliberately modify, distort or falsify this true self in self presentation to others. It may be important to nurses in their process of self-reflection to wonder when they are modifying their true selves. Do we do this when we go for a job interview or when we do interpersonal skills activities or when we write our examination questions? Do we ever try to hide our real selves?

Are we successful? Is this the basis of being a good actor? If we can present ourselves in different ways, do we have one real self? Is it a good idea to think in terms of one real self? The **actual self** has been described as the real self in the sense of behaviours, traits, individual differences or characteristics (Baumeister and Tice, 1986). There are many psychometric tests that have been devised such as intelligence scales, the 16 Personality Factor Questionnaire (Cattell *et al.*, 1970), the Eysenck Personality Questionnaire (Eysenck and Eysenck, 1975) and the Thematic Apperception Test (Murray, 1943; McClelland, 1975). It could be said that these tests give invaluable feedback on the actual self. It is because they have been devised as validated and reliable tests using norms and factor analysis, that they are capable of giving stimulus to our self-reflection. The reader is advised to try to ask local psychologists or teachers if they have these questionnaires available to use. They must be used under controlled conditions and the analysis guided by an experienced person.

Finally, there is the **ideal self**. This is the sort of person that we would like to be. It actually represents our ambitions for the perfect self. It is interesting that we never achieve our perfect self simply because imperfections are a feature of human nature. It is worth understanding the concept of ideal self because it may be that it is the formulation of a too-idealized self and that it is the size of the gap between our actual self and our ideal self that can cause the greatest self-recrimination. In this context, it is worth raising the concept of self-esteem. Self-esteem describes how we feel about our self rather than what we think about ourselves. It describes the emotions we experience when we evaluate the self. These feelings may be positive or negative and positive feelings contribute to high self-esteem, negative feelings to low self-esteem. It is believed that self-esteem can be learned and, in the context of this book, these views support the assertion that it can be considered a precursor to social skill if not a social skill in itself. A quote from one worker in the field provides an apt overview of self-esteem, "self-esteem is both conscious and unconscious. It is an ongoing evaluation of yourself. A belief of what you can and cannot do. Self-esteem can be learned! But it does not happen overnight or by chance" (Palladino, 1989).

Now try Activity 3 at the end of the chapter that will help you to begin to learn positive self esteem.

THE CHALLENGE OF THE ACTUAL SELF

It was suggested earlier that one of the ways in which we can achieve self-reflection is to match feedback about the actual self with the self-concept and the ideal self. One such technique for doing this comes from the field of geometric psychology (from Career Track International, Milton Keynes UK).

The following activity will show you five shapes. When you look at these five shapes, choose the one that you find most appealing – the one that you like the most. Accept the figure that you think of first. You cannot change your mind. Turn to the end of this chapter, page 103 and choose the shape you like best.

Geometric psychology is based on the assumption that each person is attracted to forms based on brain functioning (left or right brain dominance) and training values (acquired learning). The choice of shapes can also be reflected in choices made in our daily lives, e.g. cars, wallpaper, clothes, furniture, art etc.

It has been suggested that certain personality characteristics are associated with a 'person's shape preference'. It is worth saying that these preferences can change with time or life circumstances. It is suggested here that for the purposes of self-reflection, it is unnecessary for the reader to believe that their personality is the same as that associated with the shape but to reconsider our self-concept in the light of what could be a description of our actual selves. It may be useful to ask a close friend or relative to decide how far the chosen shape reflects your actual self.

1. The **circle** is likeable, loveable and people-oriented; looks for harmony, is nurturing and emotional, is genuine about feeling and wants to know that everyone is OK; aims to create one big happy family; is a good communicator and a good listener; is empathetic and reads people well. He or she is generally tuned in to subtle body language; tells phoney people from the genuine and is a good team member. On the other hand, the 'circle' has difficulty when becoming the boss; is uncomfortable in making unpopular decisions; is easily influenced by others and does not like conflict; is often not tough enough to get the job done.

2. The **triangle** is a natural leader, is confident, outspoken, dogmatic and ambitious; loves recognition and regards upward mobility as important; focuses energy on the goal at hand without being side-tracked; can be very decisive. On the other hand, decisions may be too swift and may lack quality. The triangle lives to tell the 'box' what to do.

3. The **box** (square) is a worker who: is highly structured, dependable, cautious, meticulous and knowledgeable; does the work but needs to know exactly what is expected of him or her; is most dependable if given good information; is ordered and must have everything in the right place at the right time. Less useful features are that he or she finds other people unstructured and may have trouble working with people; is not good at giving eye contact; can be poor at team work; has more knowledge than the other shapes but does not know what to do with it. They can be very indecisive.

4. The **rectangle**. This shape is a shape of change and all persons may temporarily prefer this shape during big changes in their lives. This shape indicates growth and transition. The person is changeable, even confused and unpredictable. It is often associated with career change. This person may be a new person every day; is most open to new learning and is in a time of adaptation.

5. The **squiggle** is: creative, excitable, chaotic, ideas-oriented and a holistic thinker; looks for new ways to do things and needs a lot of stimulation; is antithetical; takes both personal and professional risks; likes variety and new and interesting things; and hates long-term projects. On the other hand, his or her attention moves easily from one thing to another; he or she is a good initiator but with poor follow-up. He or she lives a chaotic life and sees things in a broad-based way.

Having read these descriptions it is now possible for the person to wonder what new insights into the self have been achieved. Those readers who did not do the activities first, and just carried on reading the text may now be deciding on which shape they would like to be. Which one matches the ideal self? They have probably robbed themselves of the chance of gaining some insights into actual self. At this point the reader may wish to carry out the rest of the activities at the end of this chapter.

One final issue that is worthy of consideration at this point is that of the self-fulfilling prophecy. This concept suggests that when we ourselves or others make a prediction about ourselves that we come to believe is true, then we will modify our behaviour to match this belief. The subsequent feedback on our behaviour will mean that other people will reinforce our self-concept and thus we actually become the sort of person described in the prediction. We can all probably remember times in our lives when people have consistently told us that we are, intelligent or slow to learn, clumsy or skilful, cheerful or serious. Perhaps we became these things because we believed them to be true not because we could be different. The author has met many able students who have little self esteem because they believe that they are not 'intelligent'. The barrier to their self development is their belief about themselves and not their ability. The reader must be wary of the negative self-fulfilling prophecy in his or her self-reflection.

CAN WE KNOW EVERYTHING ABOUT OURSELVES?

The simple answer to this seems to be no. Support for this assertion can be found in the work of Sigmund Freud. The tenets of his psychoanalytical school of thought have received more than their fair share of critical scrutiny. It seems, however, that one of Freud's key concepts, that of unconscious motivation, has been readily accepted by scholars in the behavioural sciences (Baron, 1992). Freud asserted that there were three levels of consciousness or awareness. The **conscious level** is the one that we can easily reflect on. It consists of our thoughts and perception. Beneath this is the **preconscious level,** which consists of memories and stored knowledge that can be relatively readily brought to mind. The **unconscious level**, however, consists of all those ideas, experiences and urges that are too disturbing for the person to keep in mind. The unconscious level can be considered to be the wastebin of the mind (Figure 4.3), a wastebin on which we must keep the lid firmly closed.

Freud, however, used clinical methods to bring back the contents of the unconscious mind into the preconscious and conscious mind. The reason he did this was because the unconscious mind contains ideas and thoughts that influence our behaviour. They leak out into our everyday lives and in some cases cause mental illness. One of his therapeutic tenets was that when the person could become aware of the repressed thoughts or experiences he or she was often in a position where he or she could begin to resolve the problem. In one

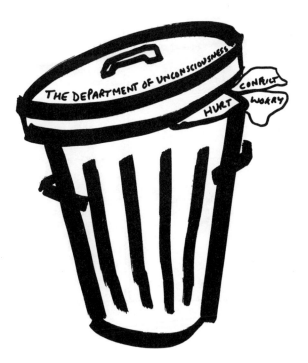

Figure 4.3 The wastebin of the mind.

sense Freud showed us that not knowing causes considerable psychological disturbance.

There is another formulation of this idea in the form of the Johari window. This will be discussed again in this book in relation to counselling. In essence there are four areas of awareness based on the knowledge the person possesses of self and the knowledge that others have of the person – the private and public self as described earlier. As Luft (1969) indicated, there may always be aspects of self that are neither known to self or others (Figure 4.4). It is the size of Quadrant 4 that indicates the degree of self-awareness and openness the person has achieved. This formulation also re-emphasizes that there are aspects of the self that are known to others but not known to ourselves. How can we let other people tell us?

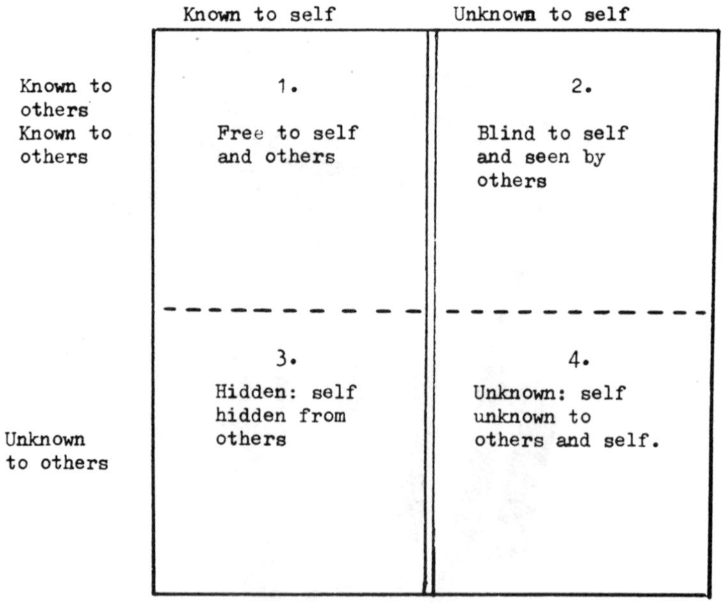

	Known to self	Unknown to self
Known to others Known to others	1. Free to self and others	2. Blind to self and seen by others
Unknown to others	3. Hidden: self hidden from others	4. Unknown: self unknown to others and self.

Figure 4.4 The Johari Window. Source: modified from Luft (1969).

CAN WE GAIN INSIGHT INTO OUR HIDDEN SELVES?

There are two aspects of Freudian theory that can help us with our self-reflection. They are the topics of mental defence mechanisms and dream analysis.

Mental defence mechanisms

Mental defence mechanisms are also called ego defence mechanisms. Ego is a word that Freud used to label the self that is presented to others. So they defend our self-concept. Everyone uses defence mechanisms, they are a usual response to the uncomfortable experiences we have in life. This is not to say that we recognize them when we are using them. After reading this, you will notice them more often. Some examples will facilitate an understanding of them. Some of the most common are repression, denial, rationalization and projection.

Repression is the process of forgetting painful experiences of thoughts. Nurses may find after they have experienced an extremely stressful incident at work that they forget many if not all of the details of the incident.

Denial is the utter rejection that something exists. One example in the author's experience is the elderly patient who had a large fungating carcinoma on the surface of one breast, denying its existence when the doctor asked how long she had this growth.

Rationalization is the common art of finding a good excuse for a weakness, a failing or a mistake. It is not uncommon to hear failed colleagues who, when inspecting the mock examination pass list, say that they knew that they would not pass because they had not done any studying, or that they did not like the teacher, or that there were too many trick questions.

The final example is **projection**, and a very interesting one for self-reflection. This occurs when we readily identify our own weaknesses and failures in other people. If I am a very autocratic ward manager I may constantly be pointing out that my deputy is too bossy. This may be some vain attempt to draw attention away from my own 'bossy' behaviour. The relevance of mental defence mechanisms to self-reflection can best be summed up by asking the reader if he or she can recognize when he or she is using them?

Dream analysis

A second contribution of psychoanalytic psychology to self-reflection is dream analysis. In simple terms, Freud argued that dreams are a form of sorting process in which experiences of the day are worked out resolved and stored in our memory. A follower of Freud called Carl Jung, however, further developed his theories and suggested that dreams should not only be seen as the psyche "as it is' but that they contain within them the "seeds for potential development and possibilities with respect to the future' (Clift and Clift, 1987). Sleep researchers argue that everyone dreams every night, regardless of whether they remember the dreams or not. Some people say that they never dream and never have. Those who remember their dreams, however, may be particularly fortunate in that they have a valuable stimulus for their self-reflection and development. It is not possible to discuss dream analysis in detail here. Only an outline will be given so that the reader can understand its contribution to self-reflection. If more is detail is required, the text by Clift and Clift (1987) is recommended. In simple terms, our dreams are usually bizarre or unreal because they are symbolic of our daily experiences and urges. They represent aspects of our unconscious mental activity.

To understand our dreams it is necessary to understand the meaning of the symbolic representations in our dreams. Those who study dreamwork suggest that there are many common symbols in dreams. For instance, the existence of animals in our dreams represent the animal instincts of the dreamer. Rooms symbolise woman as Mother. Flying dreams are related to a wish to escape from the responsibilities and pressures of everyday life. A shadow (a figure of the same sex as the dreamer) or person who the dreamer cannot recognize represents the neglected side of the individual. Going into water or returning to water represents a desire to renew strength. (Chetwyn, 1972; Coxhead and Hiller, 1976). The more enlightened approach to dream analysis does not seek to determine for the dreamer the meaning of the dream but to encourage the person to explain what they feel their own dream means. Knowledge of the symbolism of dreams is useful for self-reflection but it is most useful when its meaning is fully interpreted by the dreamer. Another piece of advice given by Chetwyn is that single dreams should not be interpreted in isolation, it is more useful to consider them in groups. A series of dreams tells a story.

THE PRESENTATION OF SELF IN SOCIAL TRANSACTIONS

The work of Eric Berne (1964) has developed from many principles of psychoanalysis. One in particular is his theory of structural analysis. This states that the person has three parts to his or her personality and each of these parts is called an ego state. The term 'ego' originates from Freud's work and is synonymous with the concept of self. Strictly speaking it is the self that we present to other people and the self that evokes particular responses in other people.

An understanding of ego states enables the nurse to understand the particular effects his or her own behaviour will have on patients/ clients and colleagues. It helps us to understand some of the motives for our own and other people's behaviour. It relates our behaviour to our own personal needs and past experiences. Before looking at the three parts of the personality it is worth remembering that the ego, in Freudian terms, is the presentation of ourselves that takes account of our primitive impulses (id) and our conscience (superego). The id, the ego and the superego are our primitive compulsions, modified self-presentation and conscience respectively. Our primitive compulsions are selfish and demand to be satisfied. Our conscience is like a 'judge and jury' that decides if our actions and thoughts are good or bad. It is what we have learned about what is right or wrong.

In the transactional analysis tradition (Berne, 1964) there are three ego states – each one representing how we have learned to respond in different stages of our lives. The **child** ego state represents ways we have learned to respond as children. It is generally demonstrated in our unmodified emotional and spontaneous responses to life. When we respond 'emotionally' then we generally display behaviour learned in our early lives. Crying, being exited, sulking, feeling embarrassed, playing games, teasing and being affectionate are examples of the child ego state. It is wrong to think of the person who is exhibiting these as being a child. It is all quite acceptable human behaviour that we learned as children and have carried over with utility into our adult lives. The **parent** ego state represents behaviour that we have acquired from our parents. They model appropriate behaviour in their influence over us and we learn ways of controlling other people from the ways in which they guided our behaviour as children and adolescents. The parent state imposes 'dos and don'ts', 'shoulds and should nots', the acceptable and unacceptable aspects of life. **Critical parents** are autocratic in the way they do this and **nurturing parents** are caring and considerate in the way they do this. When we tell other people what to do, control them or impose our wishes on them we are generally using our parent ego state. The **adult** ego state is objective and strives to be rational. The person, like a scientist is using logical steps to acquire and sort information in order to obtain solutions to the problems of life. It is unemotional and we generally call people 'sensible' who are acting in this way. Some critical points for the understanding of oneself and others are that:

1. We all adopt these ego states at various times in our transactions with others.
2. Each person has a habit of using some ego states more often than others. We all differ in the ego state that we use most often, the ego

state we are most skilled with and the ego state we use first in our transactions with other people.

3. The ego state that we display anticipates the ego state which the other person will display. There may be a match or mismatch. A mismatch will disrupt transactions and impede rapport.

4. We can each change our ego state to complement the behaviour of the other person if we wish.

This last statement indicates how reflecting on one's ego state can help to mediate interpersonal transactions.

SELF-REFLECTION AND NURSING PRACTICE

It is not appropriate to give practical hints on self-reflection in nursing practice but it may be useful to discuss the ways in which the skill and art of self-reflection may improve the quality of the reader's nursing practice. The patient is the most obvious beneficiary. How, then, can the patient benefit from the nurse's engagement in self-reflection? The first issue is that the nurse's presentation of self can have enormous impact on the patient. Patients formulate attitudes about nurses in general, hospital staff, the hospital and the health service sometimes by their initial experiences with one or two people. Since patients are often in a vulnerable state during their admission to hospital, the presentation of self can determine the stress state of each patient. Presentation of self will influence the degree of reassurance that the nurse gives to the patient (Figure 4.5). Consistency in self presentation will also determine the degree of rapport that is achieved between the nurse and the patient. The degree of rapport will also determine whether the relationship will have therapeutic effects. One example of a potential therapeutic effect arising from high rapport is that counselling will be much more effective. The nurse and the patient will establish a degree of trust and genuineness that often accelerates the process of counselling.

Another way in which the practice of self-reflection can enable the nurse to help the patient is when the patient has problems with positive self-esteem. There are many example where patients may develop poor self-esteem that may be associated with changes in self-concept and a mismatch between actual self and ideal self. Patients may suffer change of body image after amputation or surgery. Some suffer dehumanization or depersonalization as a consequence of chronic illness or mental illness. Illness is associated with major life changes and these often bring about change in the persons self-concept. Some patients are, or feel that they are stigmatized after

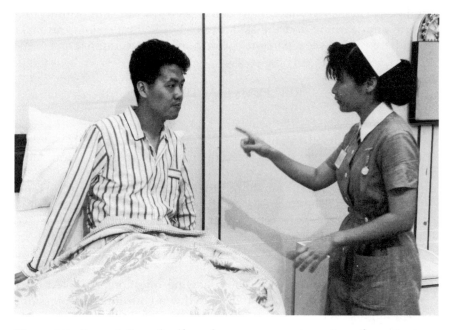

Figure 4.5 Presentation of self can have enormous impact on the patient.

illness or disease. In these cases it is possible to suggest that the nurse's experience of self-reflection and maintaining positive self-esteem can enable him or her to alleviate the patient's personal conflict. This can be done by appropriate sharing, self-esteem exercises as well as through counselling. It is also probable that the nurse can help the patient avoid the consequences of self-fulfilling prophecies.

Given that nursing is invariably carried out in collaboration with other nurses and health care professionals, it is important to see self-reflection as an important personal skill required for good teamwork. Our understanding of the effects we have on our colleagues and their feedback to us helps us to make a better contribution to teamwork and promotes team building.

It is also common for nurses to feel stress and conflict at work. This is often due to the pace and complexity of work in complex institutions like the hospital or health centre. There are also added consequences of the therapeutic use of self. Those nurses who care for (become personally involved with) their patients at even the lowest levels, may at times need to reflect on their own motives, emotions, values and behaviour. At times nurses will need to maintain their self-esteem, mediate the nature of nurse–patient relationship or justify their failures to themselves and others. Nursing work is very stimulating and rewarding but at times it can give rise to personal conflict. Personal conflict can be viewed as an opportunity for growth and learning and the skill, of positive self-reflection, can make the difference between personal growth and self-recrimination.

REFLECTIVE ACTIVITIES

1. The *'Twenty Statements'* problem. Make a list of 20 things you can say about yourself in answer to the question "Who am I?'. Do not hesitate and write down everything that comes to mind fairly spontaneously.
2. Make a list of what **you** think other people see as your personal characteristics. Then ask somebody who knows you pretty well to make up a list of **your** personal characteristics. Compare these two lists with your answers to the *'Twenty Statements'* problem. Are there differences? Are there any aspects of your friend's list you disagree with?
3. Think carefully and answer the following questions (adapted from Palladino, 1989). Be honest and write down your initial impressions or thoughts. Writing the answers down helps you to communicate with yourself.
   (a) Write three positive words that describe yourself.
   (b) What single factor contributes most to your self-esteem?
   (c) What do you consider to be your greatest accomplishment?
   (d) What would your best friend say is your most positive attribute?
   (e) What was the most positive message your parents gave to you?
   (f) What would you like to be most remembered for in your life?
4. Coat of arms (adapted from Brandes and Phillips, 1979). On a sheet of A4 paper draw a shield like the one below in Figure 4.6. Write in each compartment your response to each of the statements within them.
5. Draw a picture that represents your current situation. Ask a person who is emotionally close to you to do the same (a partner, family member or friend). Discuss your drawings
6. Take one defence mechanism, such as rationalization, and spend 1 day at work listening to other peoples 'excuses' for their behaviour. Did you use any rationalizations?
7. Keep a pencil and some notepaper by your bed for 1 week. When you wake up on a morning write down **anything** and **everything** you can remember about your dream. Some light sleepers may wake numerous times and then go back to sleep. If you do this try to make a quick note of the topic of the dream before you go off to sleep. Try to do this for 4–7 days. Looking at your weekly record try to make sense of the dreams in terms of the events in your daily life and recent life. When you have one of your dreams try to 'see' if the

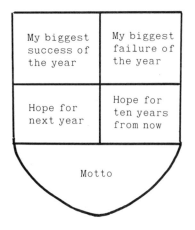

Figure 4.6 Coat of arms. Source: adapted from Brandes and Phillips (1979).

light is on or off. Try to go over to light switch and turn it on or off. Can you do this? Some people say that they can.

8. Choose the one figure from those given in Figure 4.7 that you prefer most. Read the description in the section on 'The Challenge Actual Self' and reflect on how you match up to this.

Was there a second figure that you like almost as much as your preferred figure? (Adapted from Career Track International, Milton Keynes UK.)

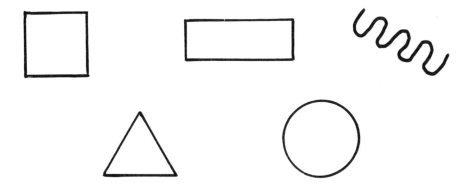

Figure 4.7 Which shape did you prefer at first sight?

SELF-EVALUATION TASKS

Take a piece of paper and answer the following questions without looking back over the text or the notes on your activities.

1. What is the basic philosophy of the humanist approach to human self-awareness?
2. Which of Zurcher's self-descriptive categories do you use the most?
3. What is the definition of public self and actual self?
4. Write down one thing you find important about your actual self and ideal self.
5. What is the preconscious level of awareness?
6. Which two theories indicate that it may not be possible to achieve total self-awareness?
7. What is the definition of a dream ?
8. List four ways in which self-reflection may facilitate the process of nursing.

CHAPTER 5

Explanation, questioning and interviewing

LEARNING OBJECTIVES

You should concentrate on being able to:

1. List four occasions in nursing practice when explanation skills are required.
2. List five common topics for explanation in nursing practice.
3. List and briefly describe eight guiding principles for explanation.
4. Apply the guiding principles when giving an explanation to a patient.
5. List and use the procedure given in this text for giving an explanation to a patient.
6. List 12 functions of questions.
7. List and briefly describe nine types of question.
8. List four actions that can be carried out when receiving questions.
9. List and use each of the principles for asking questions stated in this text.
10. Define the word 'interview' so that it reflects a variety of situations commonly referred to as interviews.
11. List the eight functions of interviews described in this text.
12. Plan an interview so that the aims of the interview are achieved without difficulty.
13. Open an interview by using the principles of set induction and the procedure described in this text.
14. Complete a questionnaire on the basis of questions asked of a patient during an interview, with a minimum of anxiety to the patient and collecting all the essential information.
15. Close an interview by using one or more of the methods described in this text.

EXPLANATION

The Need for Explanation

Much research indicates that explanation is one of the most inefficiently used social skills in nursing. Nurses, because of the amount of time they spend with the patient, are frequently best placed as providers of information. The fact that patients are unhappy about the amount of information given to them is well documented (Barnes, 1961; Raphael, 1969; Coghill, 1971; Cartwright, 1964; Ley, 1988). Spelman *et al.* (1966) found that the two greatest areas of dissatisfaction were: (i) not being told about diagnosis or prognosis; and (ii) being told nothing at all. Hayward (1975) suggests that one of the major weaknesses of information-giving in hospitals is that patients are *told*, i.e. given information by vocal means (explanation) rather than in writing. As already discussed, verbal/vocal communication is transient, so that the units of meaning are rapidly lost. Research related to explanation-giving by doctors shows that patients cannot recall much of what has been explained to them (Ley, 1988). Overall it is safe to assume that the skill of explanation is a very necessary nursing skill that needs to be more fully perfected in clinical practice (see Wilson-Barnett, in Bridge and Macleod Clark, 1981).

When to Use Explanation Skill

In order to use this skill it is necessary to be able to identify those situations in nursing practice when it can be used.

Response to Questions

Patients, learners and colleagues often ask questions, which indicates that an explanation is required. When people ask questions that seek clarification, justification, reason or just plain information, explanation can be a suitable response. Open questions tend to encourage explanation, whereas closed questions tend to discourage it. Questions from patients can have many other functions and it will be necessary for the nurse to identify the function of the question, both explicit and implicit, before he or she chooses a response. Sometimes counselling or reassurance skill will be more appropriate (Chapters 5 and 6).

Alleviating Anxiety

The influence that explanation can have as a reassuring response is discussed in more depth in the next chapter in this book. The studies of Hayward (1975) and Boore (1978) have shown the positive effects of information-giving in minimizing anxiety and the subsequent relief to pain. Elms and Leonard (1966) have also shown how explanation relieves anxiety on admission.

Gaining Co-operation

This does not mean ensuring subservience or compliance from the patient. There are many occasions when nurses must enlist the assistance of the patient when carrying out medical and nursing procedures. In fact it is difficult to conceive of attempts to do anything 'on' a conscious patient without enlisting his or her help. Patients are actually participants in all procedures carried out on them. Satisfactory explanation will ensure that the patient understands what he or she is expected to do. The success of some procedures, such as passing a nasogastric tube, can be measured almost totally by the quality of the explanation given to the patient. It is still possible to find nurses explaining after problems have occurred. It seems that we take for granted that the patient automatically knows when to swallow, when to move, when to keep still or when to say when it hurts. Explanations are sometimes attempted during the procedure, when the patient has, for example, not held his crutches properly (Figure 5.1), clutched hold of a hot inhalation bottle, touched a sterile towel or moving when he should not. Good clear explanations should be given before any aspects of the procedure have been undertaken.

Teaching Others

The contribution that explanation makes towards helping others to learn cannot be underestimated. Patients need careful explanation in several learning situations such as:

- self-administration of insulin;
- stoma care;
- cooking, dressing, bathing with physical disability;
- feeding a baby;
- changing a nappy;
- controlling aggression;
- coping with a pacemaker;
- inserting prostheses;
- physiotherapy exercises;
- use of equipment in hospital and a home.

While it will be obvious that explanations need to be given when teaching patients and nurse learners, it is rarely effective to use explanation on its own.

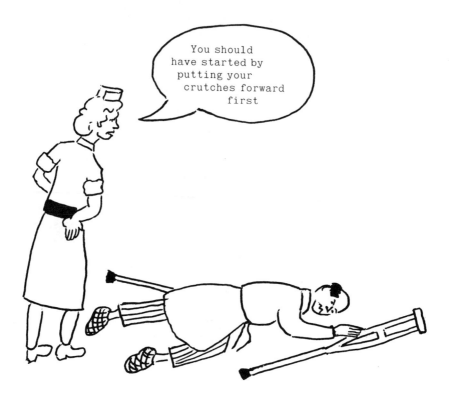

Figure 5.1 Explaining too late.

Common Topics for Explanation

The Illness and its Outcome

The studies of Parkin (1976) and Ellis *et al.*(1979) point to this as being one of the major areas of concern for the patient. Hayward (1975) suggests that technical/professional information is more difficult for patients to obtain by casual means and that there is no reason why nurses should not remedy this by formal explanation, provided that they have a competent knowledge of the procedure needing to be explained. Patients want to know the cause of symptoms, whether they will become worse and what are the likely disabling or disfiguring consequences. It is not easy for nurses to give freely all the information required by the patients, and they are frequently compelled to check how much they are allowed to explain and which explanations they are responsible for giving with senior nurses and other members of the health care team.

The Future

Here the patient is wanting to know what is going to happen during his or her stay in hospital, after the operation or when allowed to go home. Questions such as 'How long will I be in hospital?', 'How will I get home?' and 'Will the operation be painful?', indicate the patient's concern with his future. Patients are placed in a strange environment when admitted to hospital and it is natural for them to expect disturbing or dangerous surprises and to feel anxious.

What to Do

Patients need to know how they are expected to behave in many of the novel situations they encounter in hospital. This may be something as simple as how to use the shower or something more difficult like what to do during diagnostic or treatment procedures. It may be necessary to explain what the patient is allowed to do, any restrictions and even what his or her relatives can and cannot do.

What Others Have Said

Sometimes patients ask senior and junior nurses to explain what others have said to them (Knight and Field, 1981). This often occurs at the end of the consultant's ward round. The nurse may need to repeat explanations in ways that make it easier for the patient to understand. This may be louder for the deaf, in simpler language for those who use restricted code, simpler for children or repetitively for the confused or demented. It is common to have to re-explain things when the original explainer did not seek feedback. People in hospital seem reluctant to say that they do not understand for fear of seeming stupid. They do not always volunteer feedback.

Who People Are

Patients meet many different members of staff in hospital, even many different nurses in the same day (Ashworth, 1980). Patients need to know the names of staff members, what they do and even how they fit into the hospital hierarchy.

Many of these types of explanation will also need to be given to relatives and inexperienced colleagues. Perhaps less obviously explanation will also need to be given to other visitors, doctors, ancillary staff and senior nurses.

Guiding Principles for Explanation

Relevance

Explanations should be relevant to the needs of the patient. This is perhaps a simple point, but it is a common mistake to give explanations to people who do not require them. Sometimes explanations are inappropriate, where the nurses explain what they think the patients want to know rather than what they really need. It is interesting how patients can tolerate this without much objection.

Comprehension

The explanation should always be understandable, in a language that the patient can understand. Perhaps the most common difficulty here is when the English language is only poorly understood. Those speaking other languages and children at early stages of language development, may find the nurse's use of everyday English complicated. Other examples include using elaborated code with those patients who mainly use restricted code (Bernstein, 1971). Hayward (1975) has pointed to this as a particular problem in information-giving. Cartwright (1964) found that working-class people, who prefer restricted code, rather than middle-class people, who prefer elaborated code, found nurses better information-givers. This may be explained by the nurse's greater ability to communicate in restricted code. However, the aim for the nurse must be to explain in the code most acceptable to the patient.

Medical/technical language is also a source of incomprehension. Nurses should guard against the use of jargon as a means of gaining credibility or increasing their self-esteem. Sometimes the use of technical language is just habitual and nurses may not realize how difficult they are to understand, even when such simple phrases as: 'Have you moved your bowels?'; 'Have you any special dietary needs?'; 'Have you had your observations done?'; 'Your intravenous has tissued'.

An additional point related to technical terminology is the use of abbreviations. Technical abbreviations are meaningless to patients yet they are still occasionally used in nurse–patient conversations. Items such as IV, SNO, OT and BID have more than one meaning in professional use, let alone little or no meaning to the patient.

Specificity

It is a good general rule to avoid vague words or phrases in explanations. Hargie *et al.* (1987) listed some vague phrases in common use that provide some good examples of the imprecise aspects of our language. Many of their examples have been included in the list below.

- 'Type of thing';
- 'A load of. . .';
- 'Was not quite';
- 'Sometimes';
- 'Sort of thing';
- 'Often';
- 'Nearly';
- 'Probably';
- 'They say that. . .'.

It would prove a useful exercise to think of how we use these phrases in everyday language.

Sometimes vagueness is a ploy used by professionals to hide ignorance when they are put on the spot by questions that they cannot answer. Various colloquialisms such as 'waffle', 'padding' and 'claptrap' describe this tendency.

Brevity

Simply because of the limited capacity of human memory, explanations should be brief, concise and clear. The concept of sensory overload bears relevance here. This describes a situation in which there is too much information for the senses to take in and indicates that long involved explanations will not even be absorbed, let alone remembered.

Language and Speech Control

The conscious use of various features of speech can enhance the quality of the explanation given. One example is the use of the communication marker. Hargie *et al.* (1987) suggest that words such as 'first', 'finally', 'significant' and 'major' and phrases such as 'the important point to remember' and 'take note of this', serve to emphasize points made. Non-verbal emphasis can also be achieved by using 'paralinguistic' signals such as voice tone and inflection, along with prosodic signals such as pitch, stress and pause. Varying these cues can indeed change the meaning of whole groups of words (Crystal, 1969; Lyons, 1972). The control of these facets of language can assist the quality of the explanation given by emphasizing or playing down parts of speech.

Accuracy

The main point to be made here is that information given during explanation should be correct, factual and true. Hayward (1975) suggests that nurses can give information about surgical procedures provided that they have a competent knowledge of the subject. This points to a rather useful generalization, that all nursing explanations should be backed by a sound appropriate knowledge. The responsibility lies with nurses to check on the facts and keep themselves up to date. An additional source of inaccuracy can arise from the use of inference and value judgement. When nurses include their own interpretations of fact, it is possible that information may become inaccurate. Phrases such as 'I suppose that means' or 'I think' or 'It's possible that', may indicate that the nurse is going beyond the facts to express her own opinions or beliefs. These inferences may be misinformed or worthless.

Value judgements are personal estimations of worth, how good/bad, right/wrong, acceptable/unacceptable something is. The crux of the problem in expressing value judgements is that they are invariably personal points of view. The strength of personal value varies markedly between and within individuals on any given point. Imposing one's own values on patients as if they were fact can be considered an abuse of the patient's vulnerability.

A final point about the inaccuracy of information is concerned with telling the truth. There are times in nursing practice when lies are told and encouraged in the belief that they are in the best interest of the patient. Great controversy still rages over whether hospital staff should tell a patient that he is going to die. The general enlightened opinion (see Hacking, in Bridge and Macleod Clark, 1981, for a full discussion) is that the patient should be told but in practice this might not be the case. Knight and Field (1981) describe this situation vividly in a participant observation study. The investigators were not nurses or doctors and their description is not marred by the usual rationalization of medical people. The use of the word 'cyst' instead of 'malignant growth' or 'cancer' provides an example of a deceptive inaccuracy, and it demonstrates the use of jargon to tell 'white lies' in the patient's best interests. Most of the claims that this is the best way to deal with these situations are largely unsubstantiated.

The nurse should work to overcome this sort of problem if explanations are to be beneficial to the patient. Consider the effects of telling a child that an injection will not hurt; he or she then shrieks in pain as the needle is inserted. How would the dying person feel when he or she finds out that his or her relatives and the nurses he or she has trusted have been deceiving him or her to such a point that he has been unable to spend the end of his life in ways he or she would have wished? Studies of communication indicate that non-verbal communications are so poorly controlled that they can be inconsistent with spoken mistruths. Patients can readily detect these inconsistencies and they will then engage in checking behaviour to find out the truth. The concept of double-bind (R. Stevens, 1975; Bateson, 1972) is closely related to this type of incongruity and it has been found to disturb people to such an extent that it has been implicated in the causation of some fairly severe psychological effects in the long term.

Illustration

An understanding of the information presented in an explanation may be facilitated by the giving of examples that are familiar to the person receiving the explanation. The use of metaphor, simile, analogy, comparison and anecdote may help in the presentation of a clear explanation. One must be careful not to confuse patients by overusing these methods of illustration or by choosing inappropriate examples.

Feedback

When explaining, the nurse should receive feedback. This involves checking to see if the points made in the explanation are being adequately received. Feedback may be obtained from non-verbal cues such as facial expression, eye contact and gestures. They may indicate that the person understands, is paying attention, is confused or not following the explainer's train of thought. Feedback may also be achieved by intermittent verbal checks, i.e. asking questions to see if the main points have been taken. Merely asking 'Do you understand?' is usually insufficient. Specific questions about particular features of the message must be asked. This will need to be carried out in a skilled and tactful fashion so as not to insult the person receiving the explanation. Ivey and Authier (1978) give the following examples of checking comments: 'Could you repeat what I have said?'; 'How does that come across to you?' Others include: 'How would you describe what I have said?'; 'Is there anything I have said that you might find difficult to explain to somebody else such as your wife?'.

Other methods of encouraging feedback include inviting questions at frequent appropriate intervals: 'Do you want to ask about anything I have said up to now?'; 'If you don't understand anything I have said please feel free to ask.' The person can also be asked to recap by repeating what has been said at the end of the explanation. Alternatively a colleague can check later how much the person has understood. The colleague can ask the patient to explain to him the subject of the previous explanation: 'What have you been told about this electroconvulsive therapy?'; 'What do you know about the chest aspiration you are going to have?'

An Explanation Procedure

Step 1: Planning

The first step in explaining should be to think before approaching the patient, about what is going to be said. The salient points can be written down in note form to guide the explanation and ensure that nothing is forgotten. Hargie *et al.*(1987) suggest that there are at least two levels of explanation. The first level seems to be giving the plain facts, i.e. telling or describing. The second level involves the explainer in substantiating, justifying or expanding on points. It includes comparisons, generalizations beyond the specific, demonstrating relationships and links or setting points in a wider context. These two levels give a simple organizing structure for an explanation plan. The first aim should be to list the main points to be made. This may be just a single point in a simple explanation or as many as five points in a more involved one. Take, for example, an explanation about a prospective barium enema. The points may be generated as follows:

- going to X-ray department;
- people who will be present;
- guidance from radiographer;
- position on table;
- insertion of rectal tube;
- unpleasant feelings he may experience;
- how long it takes;
- what happens on return to the ward.

The next stage will involve deciding on what expansion will be necessary. What examples, analogies or illustrations will be given? One will need to consider popular misconceptions that indicate more thorough explanation. The plan should then look as follows:

1. Point 1   Expansion A
             Expansion B
2. Point 2
3. Point 3   Expansion A
             Expansion B
             Expansion C
             etc.

Where explanations are commonly reproduced for different patients it is well worth going through this planning procedure thoroughly at least once. Simpler explanations may only require reflective thought along these lines before speaking to the patient. The nurse is now ready to approach the patient.

Step 2: Checking the Patient's Knowledge

It is as well to ask the patient what he or she already knows about the topic of the proposed explanation. Patients receive information from fellow patients, relatives and friends who may have been in hospital, even other members of staff of all disciplines. Not only does checking prevent the nurse giving unnecessary information, it also gives an opportunity to tune into any misconceptions, preconceptions or fears that the patient has. Some of these can be mentally added to the plan.

Step 3: Presentation

The actual explanation is now given, guided by the plan that has been previously drawn up. The following format is suggested for the presentation of each point: (i) point; (ii) expansion; (iii) check; and (iv) clarification.

Firstly, the point to be made is clearly and directly stated: 'You will be given an injection in the back of the hand'. Then the relevant expansions are given. For example: 'This is to make you go to sleep'; 'It will feel much the same as the injection you had when the doctor took the blood sample yesterday'; 'It feels quite pleasant and it is similar to the feeling you get when you go to sleep at night'. A good example of a detailed explanation for a prospective barium enema is given by Wilson-Barnett in Bridge and Macleod Clark (1981).

A check can be made now by asking 'Is there anything you want to ask?' or 'Is that clear?' This should be followed by a suitable pause to give the patient time to collect his or her thoughts. Any questions can be answered and confusions clarified before proceeding to the next point.

Step 4: Concluding the Explanation

Three actions can be carried out at this point; summarizing, leaving a permanent reminder and planning follow-up. Summarizing involves a quick recap of the salient point. This can be carried out by nurses or they may get the patients to do this to enable them to assess the effectiveness of the explanation. Leaving a permanent reminder means leaving written notes, diagrams or explanatory text that patients can use to assist them in their recollections of the explanation. Finally an appointment can be made at a later time for the patient and nurse to meet again to clarify anything that has occurred to the patient as a result of his or her reflections on the explanation.

This explanation procedure may seem, for practical use, somewhat cumbersome at first sight. With practice, however, it will not be as time-consuming as it appears. Initial experience of practical procedures such as the medicine round or dressing technique often has the same effect. The procedure is initially slow and protracted but frequent practice causes it to appear simple and efficient. In the same way, social skill procedures such as explanation can be just as simple and practicable.

QUESTIONS AND QUESTIONING

Questions are verbal communications that initiate particular responses, verbal or non-verbal in others. A good understanding of questioning is required by the nurse to acquire two important skills: (i) dealing with questions from others; and (ii) asking questions. In order to become skilled in both of these activities it is essential to have a knowledge of the functions of questions and the types of question that may be asked.

Function of Questions

The most important point for the nurse to remember about patients' questions is that they are not always asked simply in order to receive an answer. It is a mistake simply to answer a question and ignore the underlying need being expressed by the patient. With this problem in mind we can turn to a consideration of those functions that questions are thought to achieve. The following description is adapted from Turney *et al.* (1974, 1976) and the functions have been grouped into three categories according to the major focus of each type of question. The question may be **questioner-centred**, i.e. mainly to meet the needs of the questioner; **respondent-focused**, discovering facts about the respondent or taking an interest in him or her; or may be **focused on group activity**.

Questioner-centred questions

The functions of this sort of question are to: (i) obtain information; (ii) focus attention; (iii) arouse interest or curiosity; and (iv) initiate social interaction.

Obtaining Information

This is such a common function of questioning that many of us have come to believe that it is the only function. This type of question is often brief and fairly precise and the examples below will be familiar to most practising nurses:

- 'What time does the ambulance arrive?';

- 'Who was that doctor, I've never seen him before?';
- 'What is this pink tablet for?';
- 'What is a prostate gland anyway?';
- 'What does ECT mean?';
- 'Will I have to go to my own doctor?'.

The list is endless and the reader could easily extend this list to facilitate an understanding of the variety and form information-seeking questions can take. Nurses also ask questions for this purpose when completing patient profiles and carrying out observations:

- 'Have you been in hospital before?';
- 'Are you married?';
- 'What is your date of birth?';
- 'Do you have any religious preference?'.

Focusing Attention

This usually takes the form of the introduction of a new topic or issue by the patient that he or she considers important. A beginning such as 'Yes, but what about. . .?', indicates that the patient wants to focus on another issue. This may bring about a focusing of both the questioner and the respondent's attention. The initiative comes from the questioner, indicating that it is his or her need that is of greatest importance. Some examples could be:

- 'Yes, but how am I going to get home?';
- 'It's alright arranging for the sheets to be washed but what about the smell of urine about the house?'.

Arousing Interest or Curiosity

Examples of these types of questions include:

- 'Guess what I've got?';
- 'Why should you care about my problems?';
- 'Will you have a look at my sore heels?';
- 'Is this nasogastric tube supposed to come out this far nurse?'.

It is plain to see here the power that questions have to direct or compel nurses to action. Patients often ask questions to arouse nurses' interest and to get them to do something for them.

Initiating Social Interaction

Examples include:

- 'Can I speak to you nurse?';

- 'Shall we dance?';
- 'Don't I know you from somewhere?';
- 'Would you like to join me for a cup of tea?'.

While some of these examples may not seem to be relevant to nursing (although 'Shall we dance?' may occur in various forms of recreational therapy), they demonstrate how social transaction may be initiated by asking questions. The nurse should be on the lookout for this need expressed in patients' questions – particularly in view of the finding that some patients can be socially isolated because they are unpopular (Stockwell, 1972). If the social, interactional and attention-seeking needs of people are persistently ignored then it is highly likely that they will engage in more radical and sometimes dangerous behaviour to ensure their social involvement or to gain the nurse's attention. Types of behaviour that may bring this about include hypochondriasis, suicide, practical jokes, disruptive behaviour, destructive and violent reaction or 'playing staff off' against each other.

Respondent-focused questions

The functions of this type of question include:

Identifying Difficulties and Problems

When nurses asks questions related to the assessment and evaluation stages of the nursing process they are using questions such as:

- 'Where do you feel the pain?';
- 'How severe is the pain?';
- 'How often do you get this pain?';
- 'Did you sleep at all last night?'.

These questions are often linked together in order to probe or explore problems brought up by the patient.

Ascertaining Attitudes, Opinions and Feelings of the Respondent

It is common for nurses to ask the patients how they feel and also for patients to ask nurses what they think about certain issues. For example:

- 'Do you think I should have the operation?';
- 'Would you complain or just leave it alone?';
- 'If you were me would you go to that hostel?'.

Patients sometimes enquire about the nurse's attitudes, occasionally at a fairly intimate level.

'What do you think about abortion?'
'Do you approve of sex before marriage?'.

It is worth remembering that when patients ask nurses to express their attitudes and opinions, it is possible that suggestible people will adopt these ideas as their own. This can give the nurse considerable power to influence the patient's decisions, which can be a problem, even unethical, when one considers the examples given above. Questions that invite the expression of attitudes and opinions also encourage inference and value judgement statements from the nurse. The danger of expressing value judgement has been discussed earlier.

Showing Interest in the Respondent

Showing interest in other people is probably one of the expected attributes of the nurse. This sort of question also adds to the repertoire of nursing cliché statements.

- 'How are we today then?';
- 'Are you OK?';
- 'Do you feel better now?'.

Sometimes they become so habitual that the nurse does not even wait for an answer. On the positive side, many questions are used by nurses to communicate genuine concern. In such cases, answers are not absolutely necessary, especially if they succeed in initiating social transaction. Patients sometimes show interest in the nurse by asking questions such as:

- 'You don't look very happy, has someone upset you?';
- 'You look tired, do you feel alright?';
- 'Why do you look so cheerful?'.

Other expressions of interest may take the form of questions about the nurses' origins, where they live or other aspects of their personal lives. These questions encourage self-disclosure and the nurse may become worried about this for two reasons. One is that it encourages familiarity. It is still fashionable with some nursing practitioners to discourage familiarity by stating that one should not become too involved with patient. Contrary to this is a belief that nurses can show that they are human and willing to participate in meaningful, albeit professional relationships. Professional does not mean cold, detached or aloof. It is very difficult to conceive of a helping, caring professional who does not become 'familiar' or involved, particularly when one considers the intimate nature of nursing activities. The second problem that nurses may encounter is a difficulty in answering personal questions, i.e. talking about themselves and disclosing something about themselves. Some of us find this invasive and embarrassing, and find it difficult to respond appropriately.

Creating Insight Concerning the Future (Enlightening the Respondent)

This sort of question asks the respondent to look into the future, to imagine consequences or to make predictions. There are occasions when patients make plans or decisions without considering the consequences of them. Instead of telling the person what can go wrong, it is better to get him or her to come to his own realization of the potential problems. This can be done by asking questions such as: 'What do you think may happen if. . .?'; 'How do you think your wife will react to that?'; 'What will you do if you can't persuade the doctor to. . .?'. In this situation, the patient is less likely to feel that the nurse is devaluing his or her decision or interfering with his or her plan if he or she is formulating his or her own constraints rather than having them imposed.

Assessing the Extent of the Respondent's Knowledge

This form of questioning has been touched upon in the accounts of explanation and teaching, when the nurse needs to assess how much previous knowledge the patient has. One of the basic principles of teaching is to assess previous knowledge before presenting new material. This allows the teacher to use the knowledge already possessed by the learner to facilitate learning and provide links between the old and new material. Whether it is the patient or the learner nurse who is being taught, this sort of question will also serve to check the effectiveness of teaching sessions. Questions are asked by the assessor during ward-based student and pupil nurse assessments, in order to achieve this function. Patients also ask questions to assess the nurse's knowledge, ability and skill. If the nurse has to say 'I don't know' too often, it is easy to see that the patient may lose trust and confidence in him or her.

Group-focused Questions

These function: (i) to show that group participation is expected and valued; (ii) to encourage reflection and comment on suggestions made by other group members; and (iii) to maintain the attention of group members.

Two groups are of particular interest when considering this sort of function in nursing practice. As a leader, the nurse will need to control patients in groups as well as control a ward nursing team. One may observe questions performing these functions during the ward teaching report:

- 'Nurse Smith, could you describe the main complications of closed chest drainage?';
- 'Nurse Smith has mentioned infection; can anybody say how this could be prevented?';
- 'Nurse Bloggs, can you add to Nurse Smith's suggestion that the patient will need to lay flat in bed?'.

Each of these questions provides an example of the functions described above. Which questions match which functions?

Types of Questions

Closed Questions

This type of question limits the response that can be made. The simplest form is that which allows only a 'yes' or 'no' answer. It is obvious that little extra information can be gained from this sort of question without asking another question. There are many everyday examples of occasions when a simple 'yes' or 'no' is highly effective. This form of question may be used to stop people from adding to the answer. The content for consideration and the response is dictated by the questioner. The potential effect of limiting answers in this way is often demonstrated in television and literary portrayals of the formidable courtroom cross-examiner.

Another type of closed question is the selection question (Hargie *et al.*, 1987). 'Do you want broccoli, cabbage or cauliflower?', 'Would you like to listen to the radio or watch the television?' and 'Do you want to rest in bed or sit in a chair?' all provide examples of questions that restrict the response by allowing only a few alternatives. An element of suggestion may also be detected in this form of question.

The third form of closed question can be described as the factual question. When only one correct answer is the appropriate reply the response is still restricted. Questions that ask for statements of fact, such as 'What is your date of birth?', 'How tall are you?' and 'Where is the pain?' limit the response just as much as questions like 'What is the date?', 'Who is the Prime Minister?' and 'What is the square root of nine?'. The only alternative responses to these questions are wrong answers and 'I don't know' responses. A possible fourth type of closed question is the multiple-choice question. Such questions give four possible answers and the respondent is restricted to a choice of one of these. This could be seen as a form of selection and in both cases as the number of alternatives increases so does the freedom of choice. When presented in speech form these questions can become confusing (Figure 5.2).

Open or Free-response Questions

The open question allows the respondent the freedom to answer in any way he or she wishes. This provides a useful method of revealing the respondent's own thoughts and ideas in a relatively spontaneous fashion. Open questions are generally formulated in broad terms but there are several stock starting phrases that encourage an open answer. They include:

- 'In what way. . .?';
- 'How do you see. . .?';
- 'Can you explain how you see. . .?';
- 'Could you describe your views on. . .?';
- 'What do you think about. . .?'.

Open questions are useful for eliciting attitudes, feeling and opinions. They can also be less threatening, in terms of requiring specialized knowledge, than closed questions. The open question allows self-expression and freedom for exploration of whole areas of personal information. For this reason they are particularly useful in counselling. From the questioner's point of view open questions are

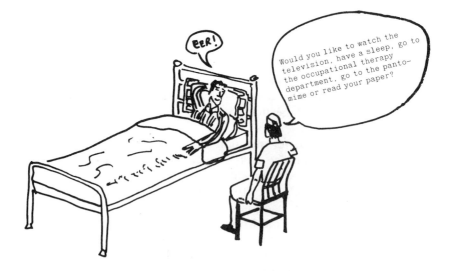

Figure 5.2 The selection question with multiple alternatives.

advantageous in that very little, if any, prior knowledge is necessary to formulate the question and much unexpected information may be precipitated. If it were not for the freedom that open questions allow, they could be threatening because they encourage self-disclosure. The respondent may, however, avoid disclosing information he or she finds embarrassing or uncomfortable.

This conversely points to a problem associated with open questions. Significant information may be missed because the respondent does not see it as significant. The respondent may not bring to awareness some aspects of an issue or he or she may embroider or fabricate certain facts. This form of fabrication does not constitute a lie because it is often unintentional. Some features of long-term memory recall may in themselves distort recollections from the past (Bartlett, 1932).

Leading Questions

The wording of leading questions tends to suggest what the answer should be. They may also indicate the questioner's preferences or attitudes. The question itself points to the preferred answer and this form of question is very influential with suggestible people or those who have no ability or inclination to formulate an answer. Hayes (1991) described four types of leading question, which are discussed below with examples from nursing practice.

Simple leads

These questions almost ask the respondent to agree with a statement in the question. For example:

- 'You don't want a bed pan yet, do you?';
- 'You will of course want the operation, won't you?';
- 'It's silly of course to worry about a stoma, isn't it?'.

It can be seen that a statement of supposed fact given before the question can have a powerful effect.

Conversational leads

These are used in everyday conversation. For example:

- 'Isn't it a lovely day';
- 'Don't you think he looks a lot better today, Mrs White?'.

Implication leads

This form of question indicates that some sort of derogatory attribute will be attached to the respondent if he chooses the wrong answer. For example:

- 'Most sensible people don't need an anaesthetic; do you?';
- 'Brave boys don't cry; you're not going to cry are you?'.

It can be seen in each case that if the person answers the question in a particular way he can be declaring that he or she is not sensible or he is cowardly.

Subtle leads

These are the questions that influence the respondent by indicating the significant attribute of the topic in question. A question such as 'How severe is the pain?' tends to encourage the belief that the feeling is severe, and the likely but meaningless answer may be 'Oh, very'. Notice how the question 'Will you tell me how the pain affects you?' differs in its likely response. A simple question such as 'How long have you been waiting?' suggests that the respondent has been waiting a long time. Imagine the situation of a complaint being made to the Sister about a nurse hurting an old gentleman while lifting him. What would be the likely effects of the following questions if Sister were to ask them when inquiring about the situation?

- 'How rough was the nurse with you?';
- 'How did the nurse make this mistake?';
- 'Was the nurse making those little twinges you get a bit worse?';
- 'Was the nurse trying to hurt you?'.

One can recognize in these questions certain influential or loaded words (Oppenheim, 1966), which are highly suggestive and are often emotionally charged. Leading questions cause problems in health care settings and should be avoided wherever possible (Enelow and Swisher, 1979).

Prestige Bias Questions

Sometimes questions are formulated in a way that encourages responses consistent with prestigious or normative values. They are similar to implication leads but the question does not state the negative value; the person does it for himself or herself:

- 'How many times do you brush your teeth a day?';
- 'Do you have a newspaper delivered every day?';
- 'How many times do you bath or shower a week?'.

Oppenheim describes approaches in answering this sort of question rather aptly by saying of the respondents:

They claim that they buy new tyres for their cars when in fact they buy retreads; they deny reading certain Sunday newspapers of dubious repute; the shirts they buy are expensive; they would seem to brush their teeth with great frequency and to visit museums almost every week.

Oppenheim, 1966

Patients will not always admit that they do not wash in the morning or that they have bought pyjamas just to come into hospital.

Double-barrelled Questions

This type of question asks about two issues in a seemingly single question. For example: 'Have you vomited or had diarrhoea?'. A question like this is inefficient because a 'yes/no' answer means that the nurse will have to check that the answer applies to both points stated in the question. It may confuse some patients or at least produce a confusing answer. **Double-negative** questions are another form of double-barrelled question but are much more confusing. It is confusing because it forces the respondent to juggle with two negative points. The questioner and the respondent may be unsure as to which of the negative points is the focus of the answer. For example:

- 'Have you forgotten not to order beans?';
- 'Would you rather not have unsweetened tea?';
- 'Is the expiry date out of date?'.

Recall/Process Questions

Recall questions (Hargie *et al.*, 1981) require relatively simple cognitive skills to be answered. Oppenheim (1966) described a similar type of question called the factual question. This form of question requires recall, remembering, recognition and usually depends on the person's memory for factual information, e.g. 'What is your telephone number?'; 'Who is the Secretary of State for health services?' It may be observed that these examples are also closed questions. Process questions require the respondent to use the more complex mental faculties in expressing attitudes, opinions or assessments, analysing or synthesizing information, making interpretations or projections. The process question commonly takes the form of an open question.

Probing Questions

This type of question encourages expansion on previously made points. Hargie *et al.*(1981) give the following types of probing question:

1. **Clarification probes:** ask the respondent to make something clear, e.g. 'Where exactly is the pain?'.
2. **Relevance probes:** ask about appropriateness of suggestions or

encourage links with other points, e.g. 'Does this occur when you eat fatty food?'.

3. **Exemplification probes:** ask for examples, e.g. 'Can you give a specific example of a time when you passed out?'.
4. **Extension probes:** ask the respondent to go beyond or extend the information given, e.g. 'Is there anything also you can say about your childhood?'.
5. **Accuracy probes:** draw attention to errors and encourage precision, e.g. 'Did you say you vomit before and after meals?'.
6. **Echo probes:** repeat the respondent's comments in a similar way to the skill of reflecting used in counselling.
7. **Non-verbal probes:** wordless but vocal cues such as 'Oh' and 'Mmm' said with the right tone of voice can infer a question. Single words such as 'Really' and 'Never' can also be uttered in question form.
8. **Consensus probes:** ask a group to come to some agreement or disagreement.

One of the questioning processes that is amenable to the use of probing is called 'funnelling'. This is useful in problem-solving interviews. The questioner goes from the general to the specific, using open questioning initially and proceeding to probing questions and then closed questions (Hayes, 1991).

Affective Questions

These questions quite simply ask the respondent to relate his or her feelings or preferences. They usually begin 'How do you feel about. . .?', 'What are your feelings about. . .?' or 'Do you prefer. . .?' The effect of open questioning for this purpose has been described earlier. One common human failing in responding to this form of question is lack of understanding of what is meant by the word 'feeling'. The nurse should learn to distinguish between two content markers in questions, 'What do you **think**?' and 'What do you **feel**?' The word think asks for interpretations of facts, opinions and beliefs, that tend towards objectivity. Questions that ask about feelings refer to emotions such as anger, sadness, happiness, apprehension, excitement, fear, jealousy and envy. It is fairly common to find people responding to factual questions by expressing feelings:

Question: 'What time did Mr Evans fall out of bed?'
Response: 'I don't like the idea of patients falling out of bed.'

The converse is also common, answering affective questions by stating fact:

Question: 'Have you been feeling sick today?'
Response: 'I've been having those little yellow tablets.'

Question: 'How do you feel about your wife having a mastectomy?'
Response: 'I think she'll manage, she's fairly tough you know.'

It is as well to remember that people do not always know what is required when affective questions are asked. In this situation the nurse will need to make the requirement of the question clear. Questions that ask about preferences, likes and dislikes are perhaps less problematic.

Rhetorical Questions

Such questions are usually statements or communication markers or they present others with questions that, in a sense, they should be asking the speaker. They are not stated with the intention of receiving an answer and the questioners usually go on to provide the answer to the question themselves, e.g. 'What then would be the consequences of a blocked catheter?. . .Three major consequences can be identified, the first being. . .' In many respects rhetorical questions are similar to phrases such as 'What you may well ask is. . .' and 'Perhaps we should ask the question. . .'.

Receiving Questions

One of the skills the nurse needs to acquire is receiving questions from others. Nurses receive questions from many sources, such as patients, relatives, learners, colleagues, other care team members and professional visitors, e.g. clergy and police. Four actions can be carried out when receiving questions: (i) listening; (ii) identification of the need; (iii) clarification; and (iv) response.

Listening

In this context means passive listening with ears open and mouth closed. This will not prove difficult as questions are comparatively short-spoken phrases. The essence of this skill is to pay attention to the actual wording, tone of voice, inflection, facial expression, gestures and direction of gaze, so that an overall impression of the underlying meaning can be gained. Sometimes questions act as smoke screens to the underlying needs. Paying attention and listening should not only be carried out but should be seen to be carried out, so that the patient or person asking the question is convinced of the nurse's willingness to receive questions both on this and on future occasions.

The identification of the need

This should be carried out covertly using the list of question functions described earlier as a mental checklist. At this point one would expect the nurse to pause for a moment's reflection, rather than giving a spontaneous response.

The identification of the underlying reason for the question

This is an inference, i.e. at best a guess. As such, **clarification** and confirmation should be sought. This may mean responding by using various probing questions. It must always be remembered that questions can serve more than one function and the nurse should look for more than one function even if they are not obvious.

Response

Once the person has confirmed a need, the nurse should **respond** to meet this need or alternatively, plan to meet the need. Appropriate responses would include:

- yes/no answer;
- information giving;
- explanation;
- conversation (social contact);
- joint problem-solving;
- counselling;
- teaching;
- reassurance;
- practical help.

The response involves choosing one of the skills described in this book in most cases. While some needs may be met immediately, others must be left for a more appropriate time or when time allows. The bathroom may not be the best place for teaching and the crowded waiting room will not be conducive to counselling. An important point at this stage is concerned with recording and reporting. Those patient needs that are precipitated by his or her questions should be communicated to other nurses by making an entry in the nursing record. Some may be so urgent that they should be reported to the senior nurse or the rest of the nursing team immediately.

Asking Questions

To ask questions efficiently it is useful to consider the following:

What function is the question to serve?

Before formulating a question the nurse should ask 'Why do I want to ask this question?'. The phrasing and presentation of the question will depend on whether one wants information, to enter into social interaction or to assess the patient's knowledge. The functions of questions should be considered here. Furthermore the nurse can ask herself whether questioning is appropriate to the particular situation.

Can the function be achieved in a more suitable way?

If information is required, the nurse should decide whether it can be obtained from a more suitable source. It can be extremely annoying to be asked the same question over and over again. This is especially likely to happen in large institutions such as hospitals. Repetition in questioning by different members of staff points to a lack of communication and a somewhat impersonal approach. Sometimes it is necessary for the nurse to ask herself how much he or she really needs the information. Questions can be embarrassing and can be irrelevant to the patient's needs. Some routines encourage nurses to ask useless questions and it is the unthinking routine approach that can cause mistakes. The nurse should always stop to consider how relevant each question is to the person being spoken to. It can be the case that questions are asked to achieve unsuitable functions. When a patient is in severe pain a question such as 'Are you OK?' will be useless if one wants to assess the patient's pain to take remedial action. This question is really an expression of concern, so why not directly express concern?' 'You seem to be extremely uncomfortable, let me help you' would be a better statement. If information gathering is the aim, one should ask a specific question about the pain.

Select the question form

This means choosing the type of question most suitable to achieving the aim and selecting the words and correct phrase structure.

Approach the patient in privacy

People do not always want their responses to questions being overheard. Besides relieving embarrassment, this will also prevent the patient becoming too inhibited in his or her responses.

Present the question clearly

The nurse will need to speak clearly, in correct plain English, loud enough for the patient to hear. In order to be sure that the other person is ready to receive the question, it may be necessary to use an appropriate communication marker, even something such as 'Can I ask you a question?' Make sure that there are no visual distractions or noises that would interfere with the patient's full attention.

Check that the question has been understood

This involves taking notice of non-verbal feedback cues. One should employ checking questions if no response is forthcoming, or if an inadequate response is given.

Rephrase

The question should be rephrased if necessary; i.e. if the question has not been understood or an inappropriate response has been made.

Allow time

Time should be allowed for the patient to collect his or her thoughts and formulate his or her answer.

INTERVIEWING

The significant part played by interviewing in nursing has been pointed out clearly by several authors. Travelbee (1966) suggests that interviewing helps nurses to obtain information, give information, teach and assess the feelings of others. A crucial area for interviewing skill is the assessment and evaluation stages of the nursing process (Jones, 1977; Kratz, 1979; Hunt and Marks-Maran, 1980; McFarlane and Castledine, 1982; Faulkner, 1985; Grohar-Murray and DiGroce, 1992). The skill is often inadequately taught and often never acquired during basic nurse training. Some nurses would say that this skill comes naturally but there is some evidence to suggest that this is incorrect. Helfer (1970) has provided evidence that indicates that the interviewing skills of medical students get worse as they become more senior. It is not unreasonable to contemplate a similar phenomenon as nurses become more senior or experienced.

This situation is exaggerated because nurses prefer to ignore the psychosocial aspects of patient care (Wooldridge *et al.*, 1968) and teaching timetables in schools of nursing have rarely included tuition in this area (Birch, 1978). A search of the books on nursing in any school of nursing library will show that discussions on interviewing skills are absent or brief. Winefield and Peay (1980) suggest that doctors need skills beyond those for normal conversation and this applies equally well to nurses. It is a well established research principle that the more experienced and trained an interviewer becomes the more reliable will be the information that is collected, especially when trained for specific information-gathering exercises (Oppenheim, 1966). As such, interviewing skill requires knowledge and constant practice to be fully developed.

The Interview Concept

There are some variations in the meaning of the word 'interview' and it will prove advantageous to examine the concept before discussing interviewing methods. The *Shorter English Dictionary* gives several definitions of the word: 'A meeting of persons face to face especially for the purpose of formal conference on some point. . . to have a personal meeting with. . . to meet together in person.' Various other facets are added by the literature on the subject, the following list giving those most commonly stated:

- an inquiry;
- a questioning exercise;
- one person is usually the subject of the meeting;
- there is a specific topic or purpose;
- a definite pattern of interaction occurs;
- the emphasis of control is with the interviewer.

All of these suggestions provide an outline of the concept of the interview. To make this even clearer the interview, for nursing purposes, will be regarded here as a face-to-face meeting between two main participants, one the subject of the interview and one the major source of inquiry and control, the interviewer. This may not serve as a good description of the interview for all possible situations but it describes the essential features of the skill to be discussed here. This allows an analysis of the particular aspects of nursing that warrant the use of interviewing skill.

Functions of Interviews

Collecting Information

The need for the interview as one of the skills for gathering information is reasonably well established (Kratz, 1979; Hunt and Marks-Maran, 1980; McFarlane and Castledine, 1982). The need for a patient profile is becoming a strong impetus to the development of interviewing skills in nursing. Interviewing should not, however, be restricted to this data-collection session. Interviewing patients to collect all new information should be a consistent feature of all nursing care. Interviewing will also be needed for information-gathering for learning and research.

Counselling

This helping skill is essentially an interview. The main aim is to assist a fellow human being to solve his or her own problems, sort out his or her worries and confusions or come to terms with various conflicts or difficulties. Counselling is generally unstructured in the sense that there is no list of previously prepared questions. The attitudes and personal involvement of the counsellor are perhaps the most distinguishing features of the counselling interview. Counselling is discussed at greater length in a later chapter of this book.

Problem-solving

The interview may be arranged with the aim of working through a particular problem, the nurse taking the initiative to move through the steps of problem-solving, focusing attention on the issues raised. Although this is similar to the counselling process, a major difference here is that the person is presenting a fairly clearly-defined problem that requires the nurse's help to arrive at a solution and carry out the remedial action.

Establishing Relationships

The interview can help the nurse to form a more useful relationship with the patient, but it would be wrong to suggest that this is the only way of achieving rapport or that this is the main function of the interview in nursing practice. All nurse–patient contacts are opportunities to enhance the relationship. Anderson (1973) pointed to the possibility that nurses do not get through to their patients very well at all. It is possible to suggest that interviewing provides an additional opportunity for the nurse and patient to get to know each other better. Crow (in Kratz, 1979) suggests that some patients actually enjoy being interviewed. This is a particularly sobering thought when one asks what efforts nurses make to meet the needs of patients for social contact.

Personality Assessment

When meeting another, one can by intention gather much information about him or her as a unique individual: his or her characteristic responses, traits and attitudes. To some extent we all make rapid assessments of other people whom we meet for the first time so that we may predict their behaviour. Personality assessment may be informal, or highly structured as in the case of interviews using questionnaires or rating scales (Oppenheim, 1966; Thorndike and Hagen, 1977).

Teaching

The interview can be used to teach (Travelbee, 1966), that is it provides a situation in which learning is directed along lines required by the interviewer. People learn at all times, not just during interviews, but the nurse can take the opportunity to help the patient to learn something that promotes his or her recovery during the interview. Senior nurses should interview learners under their supervision to facilitate learning and complete learners' reports.

Personnel Selection

This is a variation on the personality assessment theme in which a person is selected for a training programme or job. Nurses may begin to become involved in selecting people for the profession and choosing their colleagues as soon as they become first-line managers.

Performance Appraisal

This is the process of reviewing another person's achievement in work or learning performance (Grohar-Murray and DiGroce, 1992). Senior nurses may use the interview to ask learners questions in a predetermined way (gather information) specifically for the purpose of assessing the learners' skills and knowledge.

Planning the Interview

Deciding on the Approach

The first stage of planning will involve identifying the approach to be taken and the type of information required. The nurse should decide whether the topic of interest is, for example, the patient's behaviour, social history, clinical features, personal details, opinions, feelings or knowledge. This will be of importance because it dictates the type of questions to be used, the interview format and methods of recording.

There are two considerations when deciding on the type of information to be collected. The first is whether objective or subjective information is to be collected and the second whether verbal or non-verbal information will be recorded. Brown and Rutter (1978) describe the differences between objective and subjective information. Objective information is essentially factual and could be verified by checking with other sources. Name, address, previous admission, dependants, telephone number and site of pain provide some examples of objective information. Subjective information is concerned with estimations of the person's feelings (emotions and values). These are difficult to confirm by external means. Brown and Rutter (1978) describe two types of subjective material: (i) self-report of feelings ('I get terribly on edge when he is around'); and (ii) actual expressions of positive or negative feeling, shown in the words used, tone of voice, gestures, facial expressions and the like (e.g. 'I dislike that person').

The first is essentially an 'I feel' comment focusing on a particular personal experience. The second tends to be indirect in as much as the object of the feeling is the main focus and the positive or negative aspect is described rather than the actual emotion such as anger, joy or jealousy. Subjective information is not easily elicited by direct questioning (Brown and Rutter, 1978) and the process of collecting this form of information involves assessment of verbal and non-verbal cues throughout the course of the interview. According to Brown and Rutter:

> Everyone learns to recognize, more or less, accurately, kinds of emotional expression – warmth, criticism, dissatisfaction, and so on. Our intention has been to use this basic human skill and, through training, standardize such intuitive judgements.
>
> *Brown and Rutter, 1978*

Brown and Rutter also describe two measures of subjective material, one being a count of positive and negative statements and the other overall judgements based on the total interview. Collecting subjective material is achieved in two ways: (i) by asking direct questions; and (ii) by taking note of spontaneous comment. They relate the following two rules that encourage spontaneous expression of subjective material in the interview: (i) openly declare that one is interested in feelings as well as descriptions; (ii) use neutral probes in the early stage of the interview to question unclear remarks, e.g. 'How do you feel today?'.

The importance of deciding whether verbal and/or non-verbal information will be recorded has been touched on in the discussion on subjective information collection. This may be a matter of selecting the particular non-verbal cues that one will watch for and record, e.g. facial expression, eye contact, posture or gesture.

Another consideration in planning the interview is the degree of structure required to collect the required information efficiently. The interview may be highly structured, semi-structured or unstructured.

Planning a highly structured interview involves compiling a list of questions and laying them down so that they are presented in a strict order. This is usually called an interview schedule (Table 5.1). It actually looks like a questionnaire, a questionnaire to be administered orally rather than read by the respondent. An interview for this purpose would normally be unnecessary were it not for three additional requirements. One is a need, on some occasions, to allow probing so that additional unexpected or unusual information can be added. This allows a degree of flexibility and adds richness, while keeping the interview standard on different occasions for the major points to be covered. The second requirement may be to allow complicated recording systems, such as special codes or coding boxes, to be included. This may be important when computer analysis is to be used. It will be more efficient in this situation to have a trained person recording the information. The schedule may also provide an opportunity to get instructions or reminders to the interviewer to ensure standard delivery. A final requirement that may require interviewer presentation of the questionnaire is that the interviewer can reassure, motivate and clarify for the respondent where problems

Table 5.1 Hypothetical Highly Structured Patient Profile Interview Sheet

Patient Profile
1. Make conversation.
2. Ask: 'Do you mind if I ask you some personal questions which will help us to give you the help you need?'
3. Ask: 'Can you hear me well enough?'
4. If an answer is not clear, always ask: 'What?'; 'Why?'; 'Where?'; 'When?'; 'How?'; or 'Can you explain that?'

Topic	*Question Response*
Personal details	1.1 Can I check your surname?
	1.2 What are your first names?
	1.3 What is your address?
	1.4 What is your date of birth?
	1.5 Who is your nearest relative?
	1.6 Does this person know you are in hospital?
	1.7 Do you want us to inform anybody that you are in hospital? Who/Address/Tel.
	1.8 Who is the person closest to you if he/she is not your nearest relative?
	1.9 What is your telephone no.?
Social history	2.1 What is your job?
	2.2 Do you work days, nights or shifts?
	2.3 What type of accommodation do you live in?
	2.4 Who lives at home with you?

such as these would distort the information given. The interviewer can minimize anxiety by gaining rapport, keeping the person to the task in hand and rephrasing questions or explaining meanings of words where appropriate.

It becomes obvious that structure is dependent on three main factors: (i) question wording; (ii) information order; and (iii) control of the interviewer's behaviour. Highly structured interviews give questions that must be repeated exactly in a predetermined order or sequence with little recourse to variation. The explanations, introductions and even positioning and attitude of the participant may be defined exactly on the schedule. Such highly structured interviews are unlikely to be seen in nursing and are more likely to be observed while participating in research activities.

In nursing interviews, it is more likely that question wording and ordering will be left to the interviewer, to a greater or lesser extent. This form of interview has been described as the semi-structured (see Crow, in Kratz, 1979), or the non-scheduled standardized interview (Richardson *et al.*, 1965). The aim in this sort of interview plan is to provide a checklist of the areas to be covered. Order may be changed, and it may even be possible to leave some areas to be covered at a later date. Wording and question selection is left to the individual interviewer and sometimes the method of search in the topic area can be left solely to the interviewer's skill. Semi-structured interviews can be inclined towards being highly structured or alternatively towards being unstructured. An example of a semi-structured interview format that tends toward being highly structured is shown in Figure 5.3, an example of a semi-structured interview leaning towards being unstructured in Figure 5.4. The aim of the semi-structured interview plan is to ensure that the required topic areas are covered.

The final type of interview in terms of structure is the 'open-ended' or unstructured interview. In this case the interviewer is guided by one or two broad aims, the interview being carried out completely free of imposed question wording, order or instructions. The counselling interview described later in this text provides a good example of this form of interview.

It is useful to note that as the interview becomes less structured, greater experience and skill is required of the interviewer. Again counselling exemplifies this situation. Aims for open-ended nursing interviews may be: (i) to get to know the patient; (ii) to allow the patient to get to know the nurse; (iii) to gauge attitudes and opinions; (iv) to collect information about the world as the patient sees it and to solve problems. A useful approach to the open-ended interview is the inclusion of patient self-reporting and self-recording of problems. One part of the counselling interview uses this approach for making decisions about action to be taken. Crow (in Kratz, 1979) describes self-recording as a method of collecting information for the nursing

Diagnosis

Operations on present admission   date performed

Past medical history/operations

Allergies

History of present complaint

Other current health problems

SOCIAL HISTORY   Occupation

Children

Other dependants

HOUSING (House, flat – which floor, stairs,
lives alone, shares, bathroom/toilet)

Other problems at home?

Visiting problems?   Yes   No

If Yes, describe:

Care at home: Details/Names

Community Nurse

Social Worker

Social Services
(Please state
specific service)

G.P. (Name)

What patient says is the reason for admission

DIET   DAILY LIVING

Special

Food or drink dislikes

Appetite: Good   Poor

Remarks

SLEEP How many hours usually?

Sedation

Other comments

ELIMINATION

BOWELS: Any problems   Yes   No

If Yes, describe

How often are bowels opened?

Any medication?

URINARY: No problems   Incontinence
                  Nocturia   Dysuria
                  Frequency   Urgency

Remarks

FEMALE PATIENTS – MENSTRUATION

          Regular   Irregular
          Amenorrhoea   Dysmenorrhoea
          Post-Menopausal Taking the Pill

Next period due

Will need: STs   Tampons

Remarks

Figure 5.3 A semi-structured interview format leaning towards being highly structured. Source: Hunt and Marks-Maran (1980).

Personal Details: Date:
                         Time of
                         Admission:
 	
Diagnosis: Sig.
	Activities for daily living prior to
	admission:

Social history, family, occupation, housing:	
Understanding of expected outcome of illness:	Physical/psychological assessment:

Experience of illness and hospital:	Special information:
Community care prior to admission:	
Outline of planned medical care:	Problems identified:

Figure 5.4 Semi-structured/unstructured nursing history/patient profile sheet.
Source: Jean Roch, Nurse Tutor, Sheffield School of Nursing.

process. In this case, the patient completes his or her own
questionnaire. A feasible alternative is to provide the patient with a
pencil and a blank sheet of paper asking him or her to list those things
that he or she most needs help with. The subsequent interview could
build upon this list and clarify the various points made. This method

would be impractical with patients who are extremely ill, or where the patient is unlikely to appreciate his or her treatment needs and potential problems. The nurse would need to discuss these areas with the patient.

In the case of the open-ended interview the nurse will need to become proficient in spontaneous probing and question construction. Skill in beginning and ending the interview will also be particularly important. One useful way of beginning an open-ended interview is to think of a good motivating question to get things underway. Other questions can then be formulated on the basis of the patient's responses. The advantage of the open-ended interview is that both parties are free to follow new lines of thought during the interview. Points may be made that the interviewer had not previously thought of. The disadvantage of the open-ended interview is that it is likely to be highly subjective, prone to the 'halo' effect and is likely to miss some important information.

A final consideration when planning the interview format is the degree to which the interview will be directed by the interviewer. Highly structured interviews compel a highly directive approach. The type of question and the appropriate probing and interview instructions to the respondent tend to minimize his or her freedom of thought and response. Irrelevant material will be ignored, the respondent will be kept to the task and sometimes the respondent's deviation may be pointed out frankly. When planning semi-structured and open-ended interviews nurses must ask themselves how much they want to control the patient's responses. It may be that they choose to be as non-directive as possible, encouraging the patient to talk freely, listening and recording relevant information as the patient comes to it. The disadvantage here will be that it can take a long time to collect the required information, if this is the major aim of the interview. As such, nurses will need to decide how much control is necessary to collect the information required. The counselling interview tends to demonstrate the other extreme, where direction by the counsellor can be minimal, although this does not always need to be the case.

Drawing up the Plan

Once the format has been decided upon the exact questions can be written out. If a predesigned schedule is to be used the interviewer can quickly look over the questions or word them to fit the required areas in the case of a semi-structured interview. Response codes may be included, or a prewritten list of possible answers may be drawn up to save the interviewer valuable time writing down the respondent's answers. It is useful to check if the required information can be obtained from a more suitable source (Hunt and Marks-Maran, 1980), such as case notes, nursing charts, social work reports, observation and the patient's relatives. In some situations, such as with the unconscious patient, these may be the only sources of information about the patient.

The fundamental principle to follow is not to ask patients questions that are unnecessary. If a patient has been asked by others for information such as his address, it should be unnecessary for the nurse to ask these questions again. From a different point of view, if he or she has his or her jaw wired together it should not be necessary to ask of any feeding difficulties. The patient who has a hearing aid or who keeps saying 'pardon', holding a hand cupped to his or her ear, should not be asked of any hearing problems. Similarly, if a patient is too ill, partially conscious or fatigued, it may be just as easy to ask a spouse about the more mundane details.

Selecting the Environment

It is as well to decide on a suitable place for the interview well in advance. If a quiet room is unavailable or the patient is confined to bed, it may be necessary to tell other members of staff that an interview will be taking place so that they do not interrupt. A 'do not disturb' notice may be made and pinned to the screening curtains. The interview may be arranged for a particular time of the day, e.g. when other patient occupants of the room are out attending other therapeutic activities. While the ideal of privacy is not always attainable, the nurse should plan to ensure as much privacy as possible. Having personal questions asked and having to answer them in public can be most inhibiting, thus it is in the best interests of the interviewer to ensure privacy so that the patient participates fully and accuracy of information is maintained. If the nurse is to interview at the bedside, he or she should make sure that he or she has a chair to sit by the patient.

Interviewing Method

The interview method described here will be particularly related to the more structured interview. The general approach to the open-ended interview will be described in the section on counselling.

Pre-interview Preparation

This stage involves preparing the way for the interview and making the initial approach. During this stage the nurse should meet the patient and establish some initial rapport. The nurse can assess how well the patient will tolerate the interview. The severity of his or her illness will be the greatest influence here. One will also need to assess the patient's ability to hear and to speak as this will obviously affect the ease with which the interview is carried out. Both parties can come together at the chosen site and the nurse can position herself by the patient, sitting at the same level with good face-to-face eye contact. It is worth asking at this stage if the patient needs to use the toilet frequently, if any interruptions are expected (e.g. visitors or treatments) or if there is anything distracting the patient (e.g. pain). The nurse may need to give drugs that are due, change infusion bottles, aspirate nasogastric tubes or carry out observations before beginning the interview. He or she should at least ensure that the interview does not clash with too many of these potential interruptions.

Opening the Interview

The information-collection procedure can now begin. This will involve using the skill of set induction (Hargie *et al.*, 1987), which, as described earlier, involves preparing the participants in any social interaction for the function that the interaction will achieve. It is that state when 'an organism is prepared at any moment for the stimuli it is going to receive and the responses it is going to make' (Woodworth and Marquis, 1949). Hargie *et al.* describe several ways of achieving set induction in several different social situations and these are summarized below.

1. Motivational set:
   (a) Use of novel stimuli.
   (b) Posing an intriguing problem.
   (c) Making a controversial or provocative statement.
   (d) Unusual or unexpected behaviour.
2. Social set:
   (a) Initial approach of an individual.
   (b) Use of non-task comment.
   (c) Provision of 'creature comforts' (e.g. comfortable chair or drink).
3. Perceptual set:
   (a) Nature of the environment.
   (b) Personal attributes of participants.
4. Cognitive set:
   (a) Prior instructions.
   (b) Reviewing previous information.
   (c) Ascertaining expectations of the individual.

(d) Outlining functions of the interaction.

(e) Outlining goals of the forthcoming interaction.

5. Educational set:

(a) Outlining the type of information that will be presented.

Some of the above are relevant to opening the nursing interview, while others may not be. The types of set induction can be roughly matched with the two phases of the interview described up to now:

1. Pre-interview:
    (a) Social set induction.
2. Opening interview
    (a) Cognitive set induction.
    (b) Motivational set induction.

As a result of the methods of set induction described above the nurse can aim to do the following when opening the interview.

1. Tell the patient what she is going to do and what is going to happen.
2. Given reasons for the interview – say why the information is necessary.
3. Ask if the patient has any misgivings and answer questions or provide explanation.
4. Give instructions – tell the patient what he or she has to do and what is expected of him or her.
5. Check the accuracy of information already collected, if crucial (e.g. repeat name, check affected limb for surgery).
6. Gain patient's attention and willingness to participate.

Information Collection

Once the interview has been opened, the nurse can begin to ask the required questions and collect the appropriate information. Questioning technique will be of obvious importance, particularly clear phraseology, question rephrasing and probing. Once the appropriate stimuli have been presented the nurse should expect pauses and periods of silence, for the patient to collect his or her thoughts. Two important skills should also be strictly adhered to: (i) paying attention; and (ii) listening. Paying attention is not just a matter of focusing on the person and the message; it also involves communicating that one is paying attention. This encourages the patient to respond by proving the nurse's eagerness and involvement.

Once questions have been asked, passive listening will be required. The nurse should refrain from interrupting the patient by keeping quiet and should avoid adding to what the patient says. The use of paraphrasing and reflection (pp. 275–6) may prove useful when checking the response to each question. Sometimes answers may be vague, confusing or just difficult for the interviewer to understand. Probing may be necessary in order to clarify the response. The principles of reinforcement will inevitably be employed during the interview for various purposes. Reinforcement is concerned with the provision of some stimulus that encourages or discourages the repetition of a piece of behaviour. The nurse may encourage information-giving and task involvement by social reward such as smiling, head-nodding, saying 'good' or looking pleased. Flattery and positive feedback are also reinforcing. Feedback encourages the person because it lets him or her know how successful his actions are. In a similar way certain behaviour may need to be extinguished. One problem that is quite common is that the patient may stray from the point or diverge from the task in hand. Patients may take the opportunity to vent various pent-up feelings or dissatisfactions, meet social contact needs, meet self-disclosure needs or even try to get to know the nurse better. These needs interfere with the completion of the interview. It may thus be necessary to provide negative reinforcement, disapproval or deferment to enable the interview to be successful. By using reinforcement, the nurse is attempting to make sure that the patient's comments are relevant and to the point. The nurse may also use reinforcement principles to ensure the willing participation of the patient, releasing enough motivation to make sure that the interview is completed successfully. Finally, the nurse must assess the amount of fatigue exhibited by the patient. Interviews that collect much information can be very taxing and it may be that the interview needs to be discontinued if the patient becomes too tired.

During information-gathering, recording the information will be a significant activity. Before writing down responses it is advisable for the nurse to explain what he or she is doing and why. Crow (in Kratz, 1979) suggests two ploys to minimize needless patient anxiety when recording. The first is to sit facing in the same direction as the patient, with the recording sheet in such a position as to allow him or her to be able to read it (Figure 5.5). The second ploy is that the interviewer should read out aloud what is being written as it is written down.

At times, it may be necessary to record certain information after the interview has been completed and this should be performed as soon as possible. A good schedule format will allow recording to be discrete. Ticking boxes may be much less imposing than transcribing whole descriptions of the patient's actual words. A final point about recording is to record fact wherever possible. Inferences made by the interviewer should be identified as inference when recorded. When making guesses or going beyond the information given, markers should be used to indicate that the information has been tempered by the interviewer's guess or interpretation. In the same way the

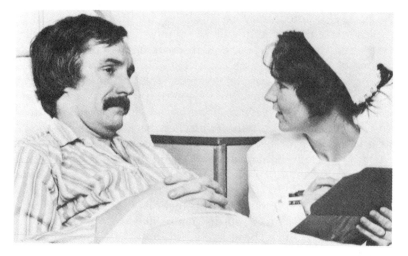

Figure 5.5 The nurse should sit to allow the patient to see what she is recording.

interviewer's value judgements should not be recorded and should not be allowed to influence the information given by the patient.

Ending the Interview

This would involve using the principles of set closure (Hargie *et al.*, 1987). All social interactions are like communication bundles that have a beginning and an end. We all learn to end social encounters by looking away, looking at the clock, walking away or saying things such as 'I really must go', 'Cheerio' and 'Is that the time?' Nurses who are interested in developing their social skills must acquire set-closure responses for a variety of social situations. Nurses become intimately involved with people at a fairly complex level and they need to be able to close many more social situations than the average person.

Ending the interview is an example of closing a functional communication interaction. Research on memory (Murdock, 1962) would suggest that people are best at remembering the beginning and end of information chains. If the interview is conceptualized as a stream of information, the opening and closing of the interview will be best remembered by the patient. The patient may form impressions about interviews, the interviewer as a person, his or her skill, attitudes and genuineness, based on the way in which the nurse begins and ends the interview. It is thus essential that nurses becomes proficient in set-closure skills so that they may communicate respect and maintain rapport. Hargie *et al.* (1981) suggest four types of set closure: (i) cognitive closure; (ii) social closure; (iii) motivational closure; and (iv)perceptual closure. Their discussion on these areas gives rise to the following suggestions for tactfully and gently ending the interview.

Receive questions

Once the schedule has been completed or the required information has been collected, the nurse should ask the patient if there are any questions he or she would like to ask. The nurse is likely to have subjected the patient to a barrage of questions and may have been strictly directive. This gives the patient an opportunity to have some control over the proceedings and allows him or her to express any apprehensions or expand on any of the points that he or she has made.

Give additional information

This merely involves answering questions or meeting expressed needs. At this stage the nurse is providing some indication that he or she has finished the task and is directing attention to the patient's needs, thus moving away from the interview setting. It is the answering of questions that begins the closure process.

Give a summary

One can summarize what has happened during the interview where appropriate. Here closure may be achieved using statements such as 'Well, we have discussed your illness, your likes and dislikes and. . .'.

State how useful the interview has been

The nurse can describe how useful the collected information will be in helping towards his or her recovery.

Interviewer's behaviour

Gathering and folding papers, changes of position and moving away, can all indicate that the interview is coming to an end.

Specifying duration of interview

In some interviews, closure may be facilitated by specifying the finishing time at the beginning of the interview, thus warning the patient that a particular time will signal the end of the interview. This may also help in keeping the patient to the point during the interview.

Non-task-related comments

Comments such as 'That's a job well done', 'That's good' or 'Now we have something to help us both', can help to point to the interviewer's departure.

Change of subject

Sometimes a total change of subject can indicate that the interview is finished. Comments such as 'It looks like it's going to be a nice day after all', 'Can I straighten your pillows?' or 'Would you like your tea now?', direct attention away from an interview setting to a different social exchange.

Personal acknowledgement

Socially acknowledging statements may be used, which encourage the patient's self-esteem: 'Thank you for your help', 'You have been extremely helpful', 'I really have enjoyed talking to you'. All these statements acknowledge the existence of the other person and his or her valuable contribution in the interaction, as well as achieving an end to the interview.

The nurse does not need to use all of these methods for closing the interview, only those that seem appropriate at the time.

Post-interview Action

Several activities can be carried out after the interview. One involves checking the accuracy of information where necessary. The interviewer should check that the recording has been carried out efficiently. One can also take time to fill in information left to be recorded when the interview is finished. Some information is extracted as a result of experience of the whole interview rather than from individual questions, e.g. subjective information, attitudes or abilities of the respondent. This information should be recorded immediately, otherwise its accuracy may be altered as a result of forgetting or stimuli impinging on the interviewer after the interview. Reflective thought and information from other sources can change one's original perception. On finding that the patient is sometimes breathless, one may say 'Come to think of it, he was breathless', when this may not have been noticeable during the interview.

One method of checking the validity of the information is to include an observer in the interview (Brown and Rutter, 1978). This would be particularly beneficial when teaching interview skills to learner nurses. The observer can carry out a separate recording of the responses and this can be checked with those of the interviewing nurse. It is best to explain to the patient why the learner is present and also obtain his or her permission for the learner to participate. Sometimes just looking back over the recorded responses may point to inconsistencies in the information given. A patient may say that his or her last admission to hospital was 5 years ago, during one part of the interview, but mention having had 'electric shock treatment' as an inpatient, at a later stage. He or she may have thought that the nurse was talking only about admission to the general hospital. If he or she received this treatment as an outpatient he or she may think that the nurse is not interested in other types of hospital treatment.

REFLECTIVE ACTIVITIES

1. Next time you expect to give an involved explanation to a patient, e.g. of a therapeutic procedure, what he or she should do during a procedure or what will happen after surgery, plan the explanation on the basis of the procedure given in this text.
2. When a person asks you a question, decide what type of question it is and which function or functions the question seems to serve.
3. Using the list of types of question, formulate a question of each type which asks about some aspect of a patient's pain. Write them out and decide the advantages and disadvantages of each question.
4. Practice question-asking with a friend. One person can act as the patient, the other as the nurse. Think of a topic of inquiry that is relevant to nursing practice. Use the principles described under the heading 'asking questions' in this text.
5. With three to five friends, plan and carry out a mock interview, aiming to select a staff nurse for the ward or department on which you are working. Two people can act as interviewers, the rest as interviewees.
6. Draw up your own questionnaire, which aims to identify a patient's major problems. Reproduce 10 of these and, with permission from your superiors, interview 10 patients so that all your questionnaires are completed properly. Limit your questions to around a dozen. When you have finished, look at your completed questionnaires and decide how you would alter your original one. Read Oppenheim (1966) if you want to do the job even better.

SELF-EVALUATION TASKS

Do not read these questions until you are sure you have learned the material in the previous section.

1. List four occasions in nursing practice when explanation skill is required.
2. List twelve functions for questions.
3. List and briefly describe nine types of question.
4. Define the word 'interview'.
5. Describe the principles of set induction and the procedure for opening an interview described in this text.

Check your answers with the text.

Reassurance

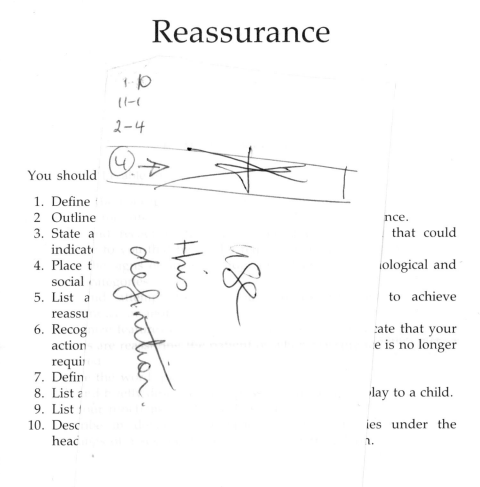

You should

1. Define
2. Outline
3. State a
   indicat
4. Place t
   social
5. List a
   reassu
6. Recog
   action
   requi
7. Defin
8. List a
9. List
10. Desc
    heac

nce.
that could
iological and
to achieve
ate that your
e is no longer

lay to a child.

ies under the
n.

Reassura of a person's confidence in himself or herself treatment situation (Gregg, 1955; Roberts, 1971; Longhorn, 1975). One might add to this restoration of confidence in his or her environment as well. Loss of confidence is most recognizable as the syndrome of anxiety, and reassurance is most frequently directed towards the alleviation of anxiety and fear.

The concept of reassurance has been maligned by some nurses as a meaningless construct. The reason seems to be that it has become a cliché, and nurses utter the words very easily without really being able to say how they achieve the state in the patient. The concept cannot be dismissed easily simply because nurses accept the concept as valid and this has been demonstrated by their persistent use of the term. A very useful concept analysis by Teasdale (1989) alerts us to the fact that the term 'reassurance' is used in different ways, all of which enable a broader understanding of the context and the skill. By undertaking a content analysis of a popular nursing journal, Teasdale (1989) identifies three ways in which the term reassurance is used:

1. Usage 1: reassurance as a state of mind.
2. Usage 2: reassurance as a purposeful attempt to restore confidence.
3. Usage 3: reassurance as an optimistic assertion.

It is argued here that the skill of reassurance is defined in terms of Usage 2 and the outcome can be defined in terms of Usage 1. It is probable that it is the constant presentation of Usage 3 by practising nurses that has caused the current cynicism in some nursing scholars. By recognizing reassurance as a skill then it is possible to view it as something to be acquired and developed, thus reducing the nurse's reliance on making meaningless optimistic assertions. The defining attributes of the concept of reassurance enable us to understand the context within which the skill can be used by the nurse. They are stated by Teasdale (1989) in the following way:

1. The patient makes an interpretation that there is some threat to his or her well-being and experiences an emotion.
2. The patient wishes to return to a state of confidence of assurance.
3. The patient achieves this state by believing that a less threatening outcome is likely.
4. That the desired outcome can be achieved in three ways:
   (a) When the person discovers the less threatening outcome by chance.
   (b) When the person actively seeks evidence of a less threatening outcome.
   (c) When another person makes a deliberate and successful attempt to confirm the possibility of a less threatening outcome.

DEFINING ANXIETY

The physiologist W.B. Cannon, in 1932, emphasized the survival value of emotions and coined the phrase 'fight-or-flight response' to describe anxiety. As such, it can be suggested that anxiety is a biological defence mechanism operating in the face of impending, actual or imaginary danger. Rycroft (1968) argues that anxiety is not a pathological phenomenon but is most often a perfectly normal reaction. He places anxiety on a continuum of emotional reactions to danger ranging from a mild state of vigilance (apprehension), to fear, panic and finally to terror, depending on the degree and imminence of danger. He describes the essence of anxiety as a 'state of alertness or preparedness to perform some action', which is brought about by a situation in which a danger, a problem, a test situation or an opportunity has been encountered, but its precise nature is as yet unknown and no effective action can yet be taken. The anxiety disappears the moment the situation is fully understood. . . . The preparedness for action is replaced by action itself.

THE INDICATORS OF ANXIETY

In order to identify those occasions in which a person needs reassurance it is necessary for the nurse to be able to identify anxiety in someone. This skill is particularly necessary when the indicators of anxiety are least obvious. The nurse will be able to spot anxiety by the recognition of certain physiological, psychological and social phenomena that are observable when the person is anxious.

The physiological response is initiated by the hypothalamus by activating the autonomic nervous system and pituitary gland on the basis of information received by the sense organs and interpreted by the brain. Mobilization of hormones from the adrenal medulla and cortex causes adrenalin and glucose to be released into the blood stream. The endocrine and nervous reaction causes several observable physiological changes. Heart activity increases and the patient may feel palpitations, the nurse may observe pounding on the surface of the patient's chest and the pulse will feel rapid. The superficial blood vessels in the skin constrict and the person may look pale. The person may appear to be breathing faster and chest movements may be more obvious. Skin may feel moist to the touch and in some cases obvious perspiration may cause clothing to become moist, especially under the arms and about the chest. Muscle tone increases to prepare the body for rapid and vigorous action and this may show as a tremor of hands or trembling voice. Blood is generally drawn from the gastrointestinal tract and the person may report 'butterflies in the stomach', lose his appetite, feel nauseous or even vomit. An increased awareness of bladder and bowel activity precipitates a wish to use the toilet for many people. From these physiological reactions various behaviours such as obvious sighing, wringing of hands and overactivity (e.g. pacing up and down) may be observed.

Psychological phenomena may be identified by personal report or by inferring them from resulting behaviour. The patient may tell the nurse about his or her feelings by direct or indirect reference to them during conversation, or the nurse may have to ask the patient about them; the nurse must make inferences about them on the basis of associated behaviour. The anxious person may report unpleasant feelings or thoughts or the nurse may infer this from serious facial expression, unchanging in the face of lighthearted comment.

Anxious people become unusually perceptive and may notice the most trivial aspects of their environment. They may look for danger in everything, thus heightening their anxiety. The patient may ask about prospective danger: 'Will it hurt?'; 'What are you going to do with that?'; 'What is going to happen in there?'. This preoccupation with external stimuli and thoughts of impending doom can cause an inability to concentrate on other activities. The person may not pay attention to what the nurse or doctor is saying, or may find it difficult to carry out occupational therapy or even remember facts such as his or her own telephone number. Anxiety does not always interfere with performance; in the milder forms it enhances performance but as it becomes more severe it interferes with performance as indicated by the Yerkes-Dobson effect shown in Figure 6.1.

The person may become more perceptive with respect to his or her bodily activities; indeed, some people may become so conscious of them and interpret various associated dangers (e.g. cancer), that they may volunteer information that borders on the hypochondriacal. The anxious person may become irritable, peculiar habits (e.g. ear scratching, ticks and leg swinging) may become exaggerated and more frequent or the individual may resort to various forms of comfort such

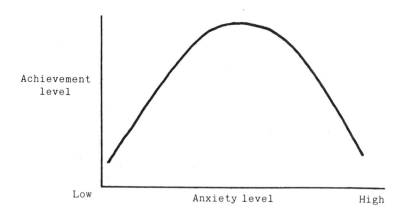

Figure 6.1 The Yerkes-Dobson effect.

as thumb-sucking (usually children), smoking or eating. More unusual reactions to anxiety may involve convulsions, fainting or the precipitation of underlying psychological disorder, e.g. hysterical reaction.

Social manifestations may include anxious people being unusually uncommunicative or noticeably over-talkative. They may be aggressive towards others as a part of the fight component of Cannon's 'fight-or-flight' response, or they may even run away, leave a procedure (e.g. jump out of a dentist's chair), the room or even the hospital.

Anxiety has been shown to cause people to withdraw from others and affiliate less (Sarnoff and Zimbardo, 1961) yet fear, it has also been suggested, causes people to group together (Schachter, 1959). Indeed, Schachter goes on to suggest that 'misery doesn't love just any kind of company, it loves miserable company'. Wrightsman (1960) showed that anxiety fell merely as a result of waiting (i.e. the passage of time) but fell more when waiting in company, regardless of whether communication with others was permitted or not. Besides being withdrawn, anxious people may also be impatient, intolerant or tactless with others.

Before looking at what the nurse should do when he or she believes a patient is anxious, one important point must be made. Most of the features of anxiety (e.g. frequency of micturition, tremor, lack of concentration and withdrawal) may be clinical features of some disorder. Anxiety must thus always be interpreted in the context of the patient's illness and his or her personality. Nothing is more annoying to some people than it being inferred that they are anxious when they are not. One example of a particular problem is the interpretation of facial expression. It has been suggested that the behaviours that indicate various emotions are indistinct from one another but are more accurately judged when supported by contextual information (Munn, 1940). This suggests that the nurse needs to make observations of the anxious person's environment and confirm the person's emotional expression by using other means such as questioning. There is some evidence that patients do not always show or express their distress. Wilson-Barnet (in Bridge and Macleod Clark, 1981), describing her own research findings, says that patients who are quietest and least expressive often experience most anxiety and depression. This is an important point to remember when assessing patient anxiety.

COMMON ANXIETIES EXPRESSED BY PATIENTS

Several authors have described factors that are cause for concern to patients. Lazarus (1966) lists six types of psychologically stressful stimuli:

1. Uncertainty about physical survival.
2. Uncertainty about maintaining one's identity.
3. Inability to control the immediate environment.
4. Pain and privation.
5. Loss of loved ones.
6. Disruption of community life.

Anderson, when assessing patients' opinions of what upsets them while in hospital, makes the following statements characteristic of patients' disturbing experiences:

> Patients get upset because they fear they can't co-operate, and they are worried about their condition. . . . Patients get upset when other patients are very ill or die. . . . Patients get upset when they make you wait unnecessarily, for instance for a national health certificate. . .when nurses are unkind, and you can't hit back.
>
> *Anderson, 1973*

Physical complaints were also common, mostly related to pain, vomiting, drugs that did not come in time, lack of rest from noise, bedpans that were cold, wet or unavailable. Others suffered emotional discomfort:

> . . . caused by boredom, communication problems, domestic worries, staff who were discourteous, other patients who were disorientated or dying, visitors who wore the patient out or did not come when expected. Many patients felt their upset originated from their own personal fears, loneliness and confusion.
>
> *Anderson, 1973*

Volicer (1974) carried out a study on patients' perceptions of stressful events associated with hospitalization. Of the 45 events stated in this study those listed below were the highest ranked:
1. Possibility of loss of function of senses (e.g. eyesight, hearing).
2. Admission for life-threatening illness.
3. Possibility of loss of an organ.
4. Anticipated bad experiences with medication.
5. Inadequate insurance to cover hospitalization.
6. Possibility of disfigurement.
7. Anticipated future loss of income as a result of illness.
8. Admission for surgery.
9. Inadequate explanation of diagnosis.
10. Undiagnosed ailment at time of admission.
11. Inadequate finances for family during hospital stay.

12. Being away from home.
13. Inadequate explanation of treatment.
14. Presence of severely ill room-mate.
15. Isolation for contagious condition.
16. Anticipated improvement in functioning.
17. Unconcerned attitude of hospital staff.
18. Spouse at home.
19. Anticipated pain or discomfort as a result of treatment.
20. Dependent children at home.

Wilson-Barnett (in Bridge and Macleod Clark, 1981) suggests that the following situations are the main sources of anxiety for patients in hospital: (i) admission; (ii) diagnostic tests; (iii) surgical operations; and (iv) discharge from hospital.

REASSURING ACTIVITIES

Wilson-Barnett (in Bridge and Macleod Clark, 1981) and Bailey and Clarke (1989) point to the need for nurses to engage in behaviour that will reassure the patient. Menzies (1960) has found that nurses often find it difficult to cope with their patients' worries and distress, and this suggests that there is an urgent need to improve skills for reassuring patients. The following discussion will involve an examination of the behaviours or actions that nurses may consciously employ to restore patient confidence. The points are taken from French (1989).

Explanation

This is the activity most often associated with the concept of reassurance, and many would believe that it is synonymous with reassurance (Valentine, 1965). However, it is only one of the methods that may be employed. It involves the provision of information about the anxiety-provoking situations and the future. It may be either carried out in response to patients' questions, which may emanate easily from the patient or may need to be precipitated by the nurse, or it may be guided by the nurse's anticipation of common fears that she has based on her past experience of similar situations. The latter may have additional advantages in that it indicates the nurse's familiarity and understanding of the patient's apprehensions but a combination of strategies is probably the best approach. Merely stating that everything will be all right is rarely sufficient.

Statements of opinion such as 'There's nothing to worry about' and 'You are doing very well' are generally thought not to be reassuring. It is more likely that they indicate a lack of concern (Hays and Larson,

1963; Parry, 1975). Hays and Larson quote Burton (1965) and Sullivan (1954) in suggesting that statements such as these make the speaker feel better but are rarely useful to the patient. Such statements may also suggest that the nurse is dismissing the problem. Parry (1975) suggests that the indication that the patient's apprehension or sensitivities do not really matter is more likely to confirm his or her belief that there is a genuine cause for concern. The reader is also referred to Wilson-Barnett (1979) for a general discussion of explanation and reassurance in response to stress in patients.

Familiarizing an Unfamiliar Situation

Here, a suggested approach is to give gradual experiences of unknown situations. A familiar example of this is the escorted tour of the ward that some nurses allow the patient on admission. Other examples could include showing rooms in which procedures or activities will take place, and an introduction to people who will be present. Role-playing of situations that the patient will experience may be useful with children, the mentally ill, mentally handicapped or physically disabled.

Introducing a Familiar Element to Unfamiliar Situations

In strange or anxiety-provoking situations it helps an individual to see familiar elements. The presence of a person known or liked is a good example. The nurse whom the patient knows best and prefers seems an obvious choice to accompany the patient to the X-ray department, operating theatre, occupational therapy or group activities. Other examples of introducing familiar elements include admitting the mother with her child and allowing the patient's personal possessions (e.g. clothing, toys, photographs, etc.) around him or her in hospital.

Touch

Evidence has been offered to suggest that human contact is a form of non-verbal communication that can provide comfort (R. Stevens, 1975; Harlow, 1950). McCorkle (1974) suggests that touch can indicate that the nurse cares about a severely ill person and has a calming effect. Jourard (1966) has shown wide cultural variations in the amount of interpersonal body contact (Chapter 3). It is important to recognize that he found that Anglo-Americans (particularly British) rarely use body contact as a form of communication. Jourard has even criticized American mental hospitals for actively discouraging touch when that may be the one thing that many patients particularly need. Many nurses may find difficulty in employing touching behaviour, such as hand-holding, and this could be positively encouraged in training such as through encounter group techniques.

Proximity (Physical Presence of the Nurse)

Even if the nurse is a stranger and does not communicate verbally, the mere presence of a fellow human being can provide reassurance when loneliness may cause more apprehension (Gregg, 1955). Monica Frost has made some pointed remarks in support of this suggestion:

> The patient remarked a few days later that she would have been unable to cope with people joining in the voices all around her. She had drawn considerable reassurance mainly from seeing that a nurse was with her and that she (the patient) did not have to reassure the staff.
>
> *Frost, 1974*

Thus by just being near the patient, the nurse can be reassuring.

Conveying Emotional Stability Using Non-verbal Communication

If the patient identifies anxiety or apprehension in the nurse, it can confirm his or her own fears or lead him or her to suspect actual danger or problems. Frost (1974) also lends support to this idea:

> Reassurance does not necessarily mean words; actions are not always imperative either. It is sufficient that a nurse can cope with her own emotions well enough to enable her to sit quietly and without tension while the patient is struggling to formulate her thoughts. . . Anyone can hand out advice, but it is the intelligent nurse who knows how to convey serenity and acceptance without saying one word. This is reassurance at its best.
>
> *Frost, 1974*

If these comments are accepted it is reasonable to suggest that proper management of the nurse's non-verbal communication will help in the skill of reassurance.

Encouraging Patients to Use their own Skills to Overcome Fear

If the patient is encouraged and allowed to use his or her own strategies to overcome his fears, this can engender in him or her the feeling that he or she has some control over the situation, instead of being a passive participant in his fate.

Communicating at all Times

It is a small but important point to make that nurses can reassure people by talking to them. This point is made particularly so that the withdrawn, the demented, the young and the unconscious will not be forgotten. One can never be sure how much these people can sense. It must be very reassuring, if you are aware but unresponsive, to find that you are not being totally ignored, particularly if you can hear while being unconscious. The nurse may find talking to unresponsive patients unrewarding, difficult or at times embarrassing in the presence of others. Yet it is a habit that can be easily achieved, once self-consciousness is controlled.

Clarification of Facts

This is similar to explanation but the emphasis is on placing the patient's knowledge of, for instance, his or her disease or prognosis in the correct perspective. Anderson (1976) suggests that providing information on the disease is a method of reassurance in removing uncertainty in the practical management of the elderly. Francis and Munjas (1968) confirm that truth, knowledge, facts or reasons are major components in the relief of anxiety. An explanation of the symptoms is clearly of value, and this is supported by Hayward (1975) who underlines the effect of information-giving on the relief of anxiety and pain.

Verbalization and Ventilation of Fears by the Patient

Lee and Sclare (1971) suggest that the verbal expression of doubts and fears by the patient is important in reassurance. When the patient must accept realities and consequences such as the loss of a limb, talking about fears can often provide some relief from emotional tension. Gregg (1955) suggests that a restoration of confidence occurs when a patient's 'mixed-up' and indecisive feelings disappear and his or her thinking becomes clearer. Wilson-Barnett and Carrigy (1978), studying emotional responses of patients on general medical wards, found that an opportunity to talk is a major factor in patients' adjustment to hospital life. Here the nurse must acquire the skill of passive and active listening. The major principle the nurse should adopt here is 'use your ears and not your mouth'. Encouragement to talk should be achieved by non-verbal cues.

Diversional Techniques

When other attempts fail to restore a patient's confidence, preoccupation with the confidence-shattering thoughts may be reduced by diverting the person's attention to external pursuits, – e.g. conversation with others, group activities, recreational activities and occupational therapy. The nurse can provide these opportunities.

Prevention is Better than Alleviation

Some aspects of the nurse's behaviour may inspire confidence and this may be seen as a preventative orientation to reassurance. They are thus worthy of mention.

Portraying the Expected Role

Patients have expectations of how nurses look and behave. It is suggested that if an individual nurse's appearance or behaviour does not fit the patient's expectations, some apprehensions will be caused in that patient. There is therefore some compulsion for nurses to conform to the conventions of a 'nurse's image'. Indeed, Lazarus (1966) and Janis (1958) provide some support for the suggestion that nurses may reduce anxiety by acting as 'potent persons' or 'danger control authorities'. The aura of the nurse's personal power can be seen as protective by the patient.

Knowledge and Competence

It is highly unlikely that patients wish to be cared for by nurses obviously lacking in knowledge. Inefficiency, incompetence and clumsiness rarely inspire confidence. The author recollects an occasion when a patient asked which nurse was to administer his daily intramuscular injection on that day; the patient showed obvious relief when the reply was Nurse Brown, rather than Nurse Green.

PLAY

Play can be defined as activity that is divorced from its objective consequences. In another sense, it can be seen as activity that has unreal consequences, in that we are allowed to do things that may not be allowed or for which we may be severely punished in real life. The child may go through the motions of killing his or her fellow child in a game of 'cops and robbers' or be really unkind to his or her spouse and children in a game of 'mums and dads'. The situation is not regarded as being real, and so he or she is saved from any serious consequences while still having the opportunity to experience, in some part, those situations. Campbell (1989) say that it has been established that higher animals have a quantity of energy left after performing all the movements required by their physiological life processes. The excess energy is used up in activity that generally has no purpose. Play or ludic activity can fulfil this purpose and may be the major way in which excess energy may be released. We tend to associate play with children but play also may be seen as a significant part of adult life.

This section deals with the provision of play activities for children and it is suggested as a nursing social skill for the following reasons:

1. Play activities often bring the nurse and the child into close interpersonal transactions, particularly in the context of reassurance.
2. When the child is ill, the nurse will need to help the child to carry out his or her play activity.
3. Play activity allows an opportunity for the nurse to observe the child's social and psychological functioning.

The nature of the nurse-child relationship would suggest that nurses need to become skilled in playing with children and in providing play activities (Figure 6.2). The important need in this relationship is mutual understanding. The child will always be in a stage of

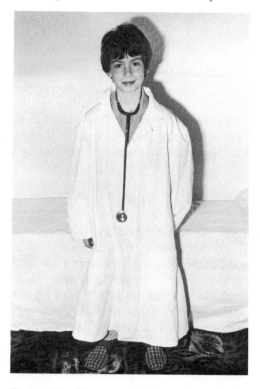

Figure 6.2   Play – a child's work.

development that differs markedly from that of the nurse. They will differ in their thinking ability, perceptual ability and behaviour. The child will have difficulty in understanding the adult nurse's mentality and this will be exaggerated by the fact that he or she is initially a stranger. Similarly, the nurse who has not experienced close relationships with children may have difficulty in understanding the child's view of the world and his or her approach to life. This may seem strange when one considers that all adults have once been children. Much of our awareness of life as a child, however, becomes distorted or forgotten through the passage of time. This possible mismatch between the nurse's understanding of the child and the child's understanding of the nurse suggests that the nurse should develop special skills for relating to children.

Functions of Play

The functions of play may be examined at two levels. The first concerns the developmental functions that have been suggested and the second looks at the ways in which play gives reassurance and helps the child to cope with life in hospital.

Developmental Functions of Play

These include:

1. Intrinsic motivation. Kahn (1971) suggests that play is often carried out simply for the inherent enjoyment and satisfaction that it gives.
2. Expending excess energy. Herbert Spencer suggests this function for play, reasoning that surplus energy causes tension (see Sandstrom, 1966).
3. Preparation for adult life. In his study of animal behaviour, Berman (1977) suggests that play, in a variety of ways, prepares the young infant to assume adult roles.
4. Learning. By imitation of group behaviour the infant is able to test out new situations and feelings. Isaacs (1930, 1933, 1968) suggests that play is 'nature's means of individual education, play is indeed a child's work'. It is the means by which he or she begins to understand his or her world and the relationship he or she has to this world (Berryman, 1991). This learning is reinforced by repetition and one can easily observe that a lot of play is repetitive.
5. Promotion of physical and mental growth. As play is an interaction with the environment, like all experience, it provides the incentive for developmental change.
6. Communication. Play affords a medium for the communication of needs to adults and peers (Kahn, 1971). It may be direct, i.e. by

personal interaction, or indirect when others observe the child's behaviour.

7. Set induction and rapport. Harvey and Hales-Tooke (1972) say that play allows children to make their first tentative social relationships outside the home. It is probable then that play has set-inducing properties and is a means of maintaining social contact.

8. Alleviating emotional conflict. Freud and Isaacs point to the fact that play helps the child to come to terms with frustrations and 'mental suffering'. It provides an outlet for tension and conflict by acting as a safety valve. The reparative effects of play have been described by Kahn (1971) and by means of recapitulation, the tension of past experiences may be reduced.

Functions of Play in Hospital

Weller (1980) suggests that participation in play:

1. Introduces normality into a strange environment.
2. Lessens the impact of pain and anxiety.
3. Allows the child to work through feelings and fears so that hospitalization can become a positive experience.
4. Yields results, recovery is faster and the inpatient stay reduced.

In addition one can consider what benefit play may be to the nurse. As a result of its set-inducing properties, it allows and encourages personal contact. It is a means of reassuring, teaching, communicating and observing. It has potential diversional properties because of its power to occupy the child's attention. It may also be used to facilitate the administration of treatment or the carrying out of investigations.

Play Provision

The nurse must assess the child's play needs and capabilities and provide play activities that are appropriate. He or she must also participate in the provision of play activity by becoming actively involved where necessary. This provides an opportunity to discuss this skill under three main headings: (i) assessment; (ii) providing play activity; and (iii) participation in play.

Assessment

In the same way as any other patient, the child will be assessed in terms of his or her personality, personal history and problems brought about by the disorder that has caused his or her hospital admission. The child's needs and capabilities for play change as he or she grows and in the context of his or her other needs and problems, the nurse must assess the child's stage of play before providing play activities. Harvey and Hales-Tooke (1972) have described five play stages based on developmental stages according to age. The five age groups of 1–12 months, 12 months–2 years, 2.5–4 years, 4–5 years and 5 years and over, represent categories of abilities and requirements that change as the child becomes older. Harvey and Hales-Tooke describe these stages in detail and list alongside each stage appropriate play activities.

A simpler way of analysing play stages is in terms of social interaction. Weller (1980) describes three stages of play using this approach: (i) solitary play; (ii) parallel play; and (iii) social play. Solitary play occurs at the earliest age up to around 2 years of age. The child plays alone, and while mother and others may be present they are ignored in terms of the play activity. When the child needs contact with mother the play activity is discontinued temporarily and resumed afterwards. Repetition is a constant feature of solitary play. In parallel play, children play alongside each other, interacting briefly but not sharing the play activity. Social play begins at around 3–4 years of age. Children share play activities and join together in groups to gain full advantage from the activity. Repetition becomes less of a characteristic feature and social interaction more obvious. The final factor on deciding which play activity to provide will be influenced by: (i) observing the child's behaviour; (ii) the child's likes/dislikes and interests; (iii) the resources and opportunities available; and (iv) the choice the child makes from the range of available activities.

Providing Play Activity

Once nurses have established a child's capabilities, interests and play stage, they can select an appropriate play activity. Weller (1980) describes seven types of play that will assist in this selection:

1. Exploratory play.
2. Energetic play.
3. Skilful play.
4. Social play.
5. Creative play.
6. Problem-solving play.
7. Hobbies and leisure pursuits (for older children, adolescents and adults).

Once the play activity has been selected, the nurse should provide an appropriate environment and the required materials. Sufficient space will be provided and the safety of the environment and equipment should be considered. One should also protect the environment from damage that may be caused by the play activity. Aprons, plastic sheeting and sensible equipment will help to prevent linen or objects becoming wet, stained or destroyed. A final consideration, particularly important in the context of hospital life, is that the nurse should provide time for play.

Participation in Play

One of the most characteristic features of play as a nursing skill will be the interpersonal interaction that takes place. This is the basis of social skill. The following points can be considered when interacting with children during play activities.

Making time

The nurse must remember that providing play activity can draw heavily on nursing time. Both Weller and Harvey and Hales-Tooke mention the importance of making time for play activity in hospital. The nurse should see play as a therapeutic activity, an observation medium and a method of gaining trust and rapport. It is an essential part of children's nursing, not something to be carried out when nursing and treatments have been completed. Indeed, play will help to achieve many nursing and treatment goals.

Counselling skills

By using counselling skills the nurse can convey genuineness and respect to the child. Sometimes children are regarded as inferior beings yet the worst mistake one can make is to underestimate a child's human potential or identity. Attention-giving, self-disclosure and immediacy may be put to good use if the nurse is to help the child to understand her and their relationship more satisfactorily.

Tolerance

The nurse will be required to tolerate two things in particular; noise and fantasy (Neill, 1961). Noise will need to be accepted but contained in some acceptable way if it interferes with the progress of other sick children. A.S. Neill, the headteacher of a rather unconventional school in his day, suggests that adults find difficulties in accepting child fantasy. The nurse can adopt Neill's view that adults should allow and share child fantasy. Kahn (1971) underlines the importance of fantasy, imagination and creativity for the child's daily living and development. Sometimes fantasy is used by the child as a means of freeing him or her from the intrusions of the adult world, thus relieving some of the pressures brought to bear in this way. While being outrageous and often disturbing to adults, child fantasy is not harmful; in fact the converse is probably true in that it promotes healthy mental development. A situation in which adults can easily participate and co-operate in child fantasy is story telling, especially when stories are created rather than reproduced from a book.

Role expansion

The traditional and commonly accepted image of the nurse may conflict with the nurse's inclination to become fully involved in a child's play. This may only be a case of being unwilling to do anything that nurses do not usually do, e.g. talking childishly, engaging in boisterous fun. The traditional nursing image can be too clinical and impersonal for children and this will need to be tempered in some way if the nurse is to participate in play activity. This attitude must also be accepted by senior nurses.

Encouraging the reluctant and shy

The nurse will need to gain rapport and trust with the child who is too reluctant and shy to participate in play.

Communication skill

The nurse will need to modify her language to suit the child's understanding and ability to use language. Younger children who are unable to use language effectively will depend on the nurse's understanding and patience. The young child will also gain much information from the nurse's non-verbal behaviour. Touch, paralinguistic verbal cues and facial expression provide the greatest amount of information to infants. (See also Jolly, in Bridge and Macleod Clark, 1981.)

Explanation and teaching skill

Children may need to carry out various skills or actions associated with the activity chosen. They may need to be taught how to use scissors, for instance, or use glue to join things together. The rules of games and how to play them provide yet another example of topics for explanation or teaching. As children imitate and identify with adult behaviour so readily, the effect of the nurse as a model must not be underestimated.

Providing novelty and variety

This is particularly necessary over a long period of time if the nurse is to eliminate loss of interest and boredom.

Working with others

The nurses must co-operate with hospital play leaders and teachers where they are employed. In addition, the parents must be encouraged to participate in play when they visit. The parents should also be invited to provide suitable play materials and to bring one or two of the child's own toys into hospital wherever this is possible. However, some clinical priorities, such as infection control, may interfere with such attempts.

CONCLUSION

It is important to remember that the actions aimed at providing reassurance to both adults and children cannot carry on aimlessly. The nurse must constantly reassess the patient's needs. As such, the nurse should carefully observe for the disappearance of the indicators of anxiety and note any changes in them. It should be borne in mind that reassuring people when they are not anxious can implant the seeds of anxiety because the person may worry why the nurse is so concerned. A re-evaluation of the anxiety or fear state should be constantly carried out and approaches changed in the light of these evaluations.

REFLECTIVE ACTIVITIES

1. Find a nurse who does not know what reassurance is, or a lay person, and at an appropriate time explain to them what re-assurance means in nursing practise. Have they understood you?
2. Go to a place such as a dentist's waiting room or a waiting area for an academic examination (a place where you know people will be anxious) and write down, after a period of observation, all the observable features that indicate anxiety in the people awaiting their fate.
3. Place all the items on the list obtained in Activity 2 under headings of physiological, psychological and social.
4. Next time you are anxious, write down all the changes you experience, i.e. body sensations, your private thoughts and feelings and your reactions to other people.
5. Next time a friend, relative or patient becomes anxious or worried try out some of the activities stated in the text or see what you can do to settle them down or help them. Try to spot how you can tell if you are having any effect.
6. When you undertake your paediatric experience or if you have the opportunity to visit a school or nursery, keep notes on the

capabilities and play preferences of children in different age groups.
7. When you next have to spend a fairly long period of time looking after a group of children, plan and provide play activities that will keep all of them occupied.

SELF-EVALUATION TASKS

Take a piece of paper and complete the following **without** looking back over the text:

1. Define 'reassurance' as a nursing concept.
2. List the signs of anxiety under headings physiological, psychological and social.
3. List the activities that a nurse can employ to attempt to reassure a patient.
4. Write an essay on one side of A4 paper on the 'signs that indicate that a person is regaining his or her confidence'.
5. List four functions of play in hospital.

Now check your answers with the text.

CHAPTER 7

Counselling skills

LEARNING OBJECTIVES

You should concentrate on being able to:

1. Write out an extended definition of the term 'counselling', incorporating all the features of the attitudinal framework described in this text.
2. List at least five situations in nursing practice where the use of counselling skills would be appropriate – preferably situations that you have experienced.
3. List the stages of Egan's Model of a systematic approach to effective helping.
4. List the skills that are beneficial for the would-be nurse counsellor to acquire.
5. Use the principles of 'attention-giving' so that the person receiving your attention will freely admit that you appeared interested.
6. Use the principles of communicating respect during a meeting with another person so that the person will freely admit that you appeared to accept him (or her) and his (or her) problem without imposing your own values and beliefs.
7. Use the principles of communicating respect in a helping relationship so that the other person will freely admit that you appeared to be honest in your wish to help him or her.
8. Formulate and use utterances that reflect, paraphrase and summarize a person's comments so that they encourage him or her to clarify what he or she said.
9. Display a questioning technique that is calculated, helpful and facilitative.
10. Describe the ways in which resistance, defence mechanism and silence influence the counselling process.
11. Challenge discrepancies, distortions and smoke-screens in another person's descriptions with positive intent and without making him or her feel uncomfortable or threatened.

12. Disclose something private and personal about yourself that is relevant to the person's counselling issue, helpful and does not detract from his or her concerns.
13. Describe what is happening between yourself and another person in an interpersonal transaction so that both parties can more fully understand what is happening in the transaction.
14. Formulate and state personal goals and objectives.
15. Engage in a reflective decision-making process.
16. Carry out a balance-sheet analysis so that you can identify actions that facilitate or hinder the resolution of a problem.
17. Maintain confidentiality while maintaining rapport and physical and emotional safety for the client and yourself.

COUNSELLING SKILL

Counselling involves a complex collection of social skills that can be combined to help a fellow human being. It is probably best to see counselling as a sequence or series of stages that a helper and someone being helped (a 'helpee') go through, each using particular social skills with the specific aim of helping the helpee to help himself or herself. Hopson (1981) gives the following definition:

> . . . helping someone to explore a problem, clarify conflicting issues and discover alternative ways of dealing with it, so that they can decide what to do about it; that is helping people to help themselves.
>
> *Hopson, 1981*

An important influence on counselling development is the humanist perspective of psychology. This generally considers that each human being has within them the potential to understand and deal with their own problems. Since we are gregarious in nature we often need other people to help us to achieve this potential. The basis of helping and caring is that psychological or physical healing can be promoted by transactions with other people.

Several assumptions and propositions are important in the understanding of the counselling process and these also form an attitudinal framework on the basis of which one can use the counselling skill:

1. Social skills are an integral part of the counselling process and an experienced, knowledgeable nurse will be more able to help others.
2. Counselling is not a mystical process, it is a skill that can be acquired and needs continual development.
3. Counselling does not deal only with unusual events or psycho-pathological problems; it can be used for everyday problems.

4. Counselling involves the formation of trusting and open relation-ship. It is a sharing between two people and cannot occur without rapport.

The following propositions come from the writing of Carl Rogers (1951):

1. Counselling is concerned with a humanistic approach to helping by increasing self understanding, awareness and the expression of feeling.
2. Counselling is non-directive and seeks to encourage the client to formulate his or her own awareness of the pattern of his or her life and experience in his or her own way, the therapist adopting an accepting, non-critical attitude and helping by reflecting the client's own responses.
3. The client does not react to reality as others see it but of his or her own perceptions of reality. No person can know the client's thoughts and feelings as well as the client himself or herself, the client's own internal frame of reference being the best context in which to understand his or her behaviour. In order to understand others, it is necessary to know more about the self and *vice versa*.
4. Each human being has within the skills and capability to change his or her life and rectify his or her own problems.

The following propositions come from the work of Carkhuff (1969).

1. All interpersonal processes may have constructive or destructive consequences (our motto to the preface of this book!). As such, counselling may be for better or for worse, especially when performed by the inexperienced or unskilled.
2. All effective interpersonal processes share a common core of conditions conducive to facilitating human experiences. One of the consequences of this is that when a 'helper functions at a high level the helpee will demonstrate constructive change; if the helper functions at a low level, particularly at a level significantly lower than the helpee, the helpee will demonstrate deteriorative change'. Level of functioning is thus concerned with the degree of effectiveness achieved by the counsellor as she deploys the skills of counselling.

The following points originate from the work of Egan (1975):

1. All human interactions can be conceptualized from the viewpoint of the social influence process. As soon as I involve myself with my fellow human beings, I become one who influences and one who is being influenced (Berscheid and Walster, 1969; Gergen, 1969; Kelman, 1967; Zimbardo and Ebbesen 1970).

2. A working model of helping or counselling is fundamental to the counselling process and increases its reliability. This predicts the subsequent discussion on counselling in suggesting that a practical process or series of discrete tried and tested steps should be identified and followed in the helping process. It should be a procedure and not a haphazard encounter.

The following points originate from the work of Egan (1990):

1. The effective helper not only helps clients to manage problems and develop unused resources and opportunities but also, at least indirectly, helps the clients learn a process for managing their concerns better. We need to find more effective ways of helping the clients own the helping process.
2. Helpers are effective to the degree that their clients, through client–helper interactions, are in a better position to manage their problems situations and/or develop the unused resources and opportunities of their lives more effectively.

To summarize, nurses, in order to counsel their patients, must understand themselves and others, must become experienced in social skills and carry out a working counselling procedure in the context of a trusting open relationship that is non-directive, increasing the patient's self-understanding, awareness and expression of feeling, from the point of view of that person's conception of reality. Nurses must acknowledge the patient's intrinsic potential to help himself or herself, and even help the patient to learn the process of helping so that he or she can be empowered to help himself or herself. It must be borne in mind that things may be improved or made worse and that the level of ability, involvement and interest of the nurse will determine the effectiveness of counselling.

USES FOR COUNSELLING IN NURSING

The counselling process may be put to several uses in nursing practice. It may be therapeutic, i.e. it may act as a therapy in the case of psychopathological problems. The psychiatric or community nurse may more often meet these problems. Coping with hallucinations, delusions, aggression, personality problems, mood disturbance and emotional tension may call upon the skills of counselling. It is necessary in the therapeutic use of counselling for psychological disturbances that the helper should be highly skilled in these situations so that occurrences such as abreaction, transference and resistance may be adequately dealt with. One should not presume that counselling is only of use for 'psychiatric' problems. The therapeutic use of counselling in stoma management, after care of mastectomy and care of the dying demonstrates the potential for counselling as a therapeutic technique for a whole range of serious health issues.

There are, however, different levels of helping that require different levels of skill. The level of skill depends on the intensity of the problem. At the lowest levels a counselling 'attitude' can be adopted to help friends and relatives make choices in their lives. We often talk to other people when we want to make a decision. Should I buy a new car? Where should I go on holiday? Should I enrol for a course with the University?

These are all decisions we may share with other people. There are, however, many times when the decisions we wish to make cause us great concern and stress. Should I change my job? How can I pay off my overdraft at the bank? How can I tell my boyfriend I am pregnant? These situations require more confidence and skill from the helper. Other issues like bereavement (e.g. divorce, death, financial ruin, examination failure) or life crises (e.g. natural catastrophes, major accidents, harmful negligence, illness, disease) require help from people experienced and skilled in counselling for these issues. Depending on their skills, nurses can be involved in counselling at several different levels. Firstly, a nurse may act as a **lay counsellor**, in which he or she uses some counselling principles or skills in his or her daily life and work. Secondly, a nurse may be a **semi-professional counsellor** who uses a working model of counselling to help with some of the problems with her patients and colleagues. Finally, there is the **professional counsellor** who engages in counselling as a full-time activity and develops sophisticated and sometimes specialist skills to deal with quite profound human problems. It is quite common for the nurse to work toward being a semi-professional counsellor and rarely he or she will be given roles that require the skills of a professional counsellor.

Often people enter into a counselling relationship to solve a problem or some perplexity. In this context, it may be seen as a decision-making process. Some solution to the problem is the person's aim. Patients will often require a nurse counsellor for this purpose. The nurse will act as a mirror, a sounding board, from which the patient can bounce his or her ideas. Sometimes the person will not recognize that there is a problem, may not know the nature of the problem or may not know what to do about it. The nurse counsellor can help with each of these difficulties.

It has also been suggested that counselling helps the person to change. Egan's model, which will be presented in this chapter, is called a developmental model of counselling, since we are helping others to grow and to organize themselves. As such we can see that counselling can help patients to learn about themselves, about others and very importantly about the nurse. This leads to another use for counselling in nursing practise, that is the strengthening of the relationship between the nurse and the patient. The good nurse counsellor will be open, allowing the patient to get to know him or her personally. The nurse will accept the patient for the person that he or she is and acknowledge his or her worth and personal strengths and weaknesses. The way in which the nurse shows genuine caring, honesty and understanding will communicate to the patient much about the nurse as a person.

Finally, it is often the case that people give vent to their emotional tensions in counselling situations. It is not uncommon for the patient to talk continuously for an hour or more to a nurse who simply listens. The nurse can be quite surprised to hear the patient thank him or her for helping so much when the nurse thought that he or she was doing very little. Perhaps a trouble shared is a trouble halved. Counselling can be a situation for off-loading frustration or boredom.

WHEN TO COUNSEL

It has been suggested previously that one of the crucial aspects of skill learning is to know when to begin to use the skill. If the nurse is a semi-professional counsellor he or she must recognize the times to consciously adopt a model for counselling in the context of all of the other daily activities encountered. Counselling can be inappropriate for some situations and equally it can be tragic to miss a subtle signal from the patient that counselling would help. Counselling is obviously appropriate when the patient approaches the nurse saying that he needs help with a problem or that he or she is troubled.

Patients, however, do not always come straight out with comments that indicate that counselling is necessary. Very often they do not know that they are appealing for help. They may be waiting to see if the nurse has time or the interest to listen. The patient may drop hints during the course of a conversation. If very little time is available, the patient will not have time to drop such hints. The person may be too self conscious of embarrassed about the problem. Sometimes patients may ask inappropriate questions or they may not seem to be paying attention to the nurse's answers to such questions. This indicates that an answer is not the purpose of the question. On other occasions, the patient will indicate that he or she is distressed by his or her body language (e.g. facial expression, posture, over activity).

The nurse must quickly decide if other helping responses are more appropriate such as explanation, reassurance, advice, practical help, social contact or just conversation. The patient will become frustrated in these circumstances if the nurse begins a counselling process, so it will be necessary for the nurses to subtly probe for indications of problems or emotional upset. It is usually best to listen quite passively at this stage until it becomes obvious what the patient requires. If conversation is required the patient will engage in turn-taking behaviour and encourage the nurse to talk. Or the patient may ask for some advice: 'What would you do. . .?','What do you think. . .?'. Questions such as these may indicate that information or explanation is really required. If the patient shows signs of requiring skills to help with problems, worries, confusion, distress, then a counselling process may be undertaken. Once the nurse becomes fully familiar with the propositions stated earlier and forms the counselling attitude indicated in these propositions, needs for counselling will easily be detected because they will be seen to be drawing on that attitudinal climate.

Counselling should be carried out as soon as possible once the need has been identified. Several constraints in nursing practice may spoil attempts to counsel immediately. Lack of time, pressure of work, inappropriate setting, attitudes of superiors, clinical values and priorities are just a few of the many constraints of busy nursing practice.

Counselling is not always seen as a nursing skill and more legitimate procedures and skills often take precedence. A medical/ technical model of nursing tends to emphasize the importance of clinical procedures and treatments. In addition, many nursing activities are carried out in the context of an institution, this tends to impose routine and concentrates on task completion to ensure the efficient working of the institution. Institutions are norm-setting agencies and they are generally ill-equipped to cope with the extraordinary needs of individuals. In this situation, the nurse may not be able stop immediately to engage in a potentially long helping process such as counselling. This is not enhanced by colleagues or senior nurses who have not acquired counselling skills or attitudinal frameworks. It must be restated, however, that one of the major tenets of this book is that the psychosocial needs of patients are paramount to their recovery and neglect of them leads to more work for the nurse not less. Counselling is just as important as tepid sponging, physical observations, oral toilet, intramuscular injection or enema. Counselling should be planned and carried out as soon as possible and not just when there is a free moment. On some occasions waiting can be catastrophic, (e.g. suicide) but generally it reaffirms the patients' belief that we do not have time for them as human beings.

Occasionally a nurse may avoid counselling because he or she thinks that someone else should be doing it, such as the senior nurse, the doctor or the social worker. One should always consider that it is a privilege to be asked to share a person's thought, emotions and problems. People do not just ask anybody to give this sort of help and it will often be the case that the person has chosen a particular nurse for particular reasons. So when chosen, a preference has been shown by the patient and referral can be seen as a sign of rejection and this does not enhance rapport. A further constraint on counselling in the hospital or clinic setting is lack of privacy. Sometimes the accommodation is unsuitable or the design is not conducive to privacy. Problems are compounded whenever patients are bed-bound, because they cannot move to a more private room. Screens in shared rooms may provide privacy in a visual sense but they do not screen conversation. Often the patient can be taken to a more private part of the ward in a wheelchair and the possibility of moving the bed should not be overlooked. A room should be made available in every ward or health centre for private personal conversations. There should be a sign that clearly says 'Do not disturb' and should not be an area that staff must constantly use. Staff will go to and fro or just pop in for something, even apologizing in the process but still interrupting nevertheless.

Finally, one should remember that counselling can be a tiring process for both the counsellor and client. If patients are too ill to concentrate or speak for long periods the enthusiastic nurse counsellor should remember that her application of a counselling model can be too tiresome.

THE COUNSELLING PROCESS

The procedure described here is heavily influenced by Gerard Egan's (1990) developmental model for systematic helping and interpersonal relating described in his text *The Skilled Helper: A Systematic Approach to Effective Helping*.

Before looking at the model of helping it is useful to realize how the counselling process influences both the private and public knowledge of both the client and the counsellor. A useful model to help us understand this has already been introduced in an earlier chapter on self-reflection. The Johari Window (Luft, 1969; Figure 4.4) was used to demonstrate aspects of self-awareness and self-disclosure. Here, the issue for counselling is the amount of self-acceptance and disclosure that occurs between two parties the client and the counsellor. The Johari Window tries to help us to understand that there is an interplay between the amount of understanding that the person has about themselves and the amount of understanding that another person has about him or her. The aim of counselling is to increase the client's understanding of themselves and the counsellor's understanding of the client. Understanding of oneself is not just a process of knowing it is also a process of accepting the **actual self**. The process of self-acceptance requires a lot of personal energy and sometimes time to adapt. It also requires support from the counsellor in the form of unconditional positive psychological strokes. This means that the process of counselling involves gentle self-reflection and disclosure. At the same time the counsellor is involved in a similar process in reflecting on his or her own helping skill. In terms of the Johari Window, an effective helping relationship that develops self-awareness, will move the double line on the figure to make Quadrants 2 and 4 smaller (Figure 7.1).

As the client shares more with the counsellor the horizontal bar of the Johari Window will be lowered (Figure 7.2).

If both self-disclosure and self-acceptance occur during counselling then the understanding restricted to Quadrant 4 will be minimized. When this has occurred the nurse is in a very privileged position; as he or she may have arrived at understandings about the patient that the patient may not even have known before the counselling session. It will also be certain that the counsellor will have acquired greater understanding of himself or herself as well as give away aspects of his or her **actual self** to the client. It is easy to come to the conclusion that counselling is a shared learning process for both the counsellor and the client, although the therapeutic effect should be focused on the client or the process may become very confusing. It is because of this that nurse counsellors should generally have high self-esteem, be aware of their actual selves and be relatively free from personal conflict. Otherwise the nurse counsellor may benefit from the sharing more than the patient. Several other points about counselling emanate from an examination of the Johari Window. Self-disclosure and self-acceptance are minimized if the person feels anxious or threatened. When this occurs we would expect to see Quadrant 1 of the Johari Window to become small and it indicates that communication in the counselling situation is ineffective or meaningless. The degree of trust that the patient has for the nurse counsellor may be low. Skills of reassurance may also play a part in the process if this occurs. The patient may be frightened of the unknown or of disclosing some embarrassing secret. Equally the nurse counsellor may be frightened of delving into a person's private life or of the consequences that this imposition may bring. It seems that all people have certain misgivings when they enter a counselling relationship. Brammer (1973) lists six of these misgivings and they are:

1. It is not easy to receive help.
2. It is difficult to commit oneself to change.
3. It is difficult to submit to the influence of a helper – help is a threat to esteem, integrity and independence.

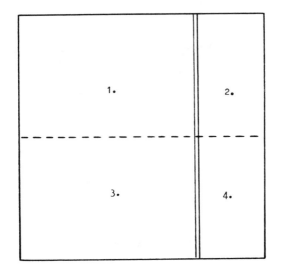

Figure 7.1 Client self-awareness.

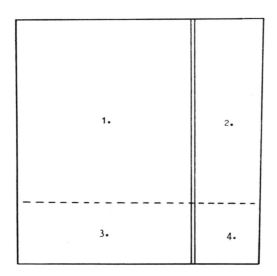

Figure 7.2 Client self-disclosure and self-awareness.

4. It is not easy to trust a stranger and be open with him or her.
5. It is not easy to see one's problem clearly at first.
6. Sometimes problems seem too large, too overwhelming or too unique to share easily.

It is important that both parties develop a trusting relationship and in the nursing context this may happen both within and outside the counselling process. A final point is that one should always respect the desires of the patient/client to keep aspects of the hidden areas (Quadrants 2–4) to themselves. The Freudian theory of unconscious motivation and mental defence mechanisms (Chapter 4) encourages one to remember that repression of the darkest parts of our lives is necessary for our mental health. Pushing too hard and too quickly into the hidden domain will do more harm than good to the patient and the nurse. In a trusting climate, patients will disclose themselves when they are ready. Patience is a virtue in counselling.

THE STAGES

Egan describes three stages through which the client and counsellor can move in effective counselling process:

1. Stage I:
   (a) Exploring the present scenario.
   (b) Identifying and clarifying problems, situations and unused opportunities.
2. Stage II:
   (a) Developing the preferred scenario.
   (b) Developing goals, objectives, or agendas based on an action oriented understanding of the problem situation.
3. Stage III:
   (a) Formulating strategies and plans.
   (b) Developing actions strategies for accomplishing goals, i.e. for getting from the current to the preferred scenario.

In this description a scenario can best be thought of as the life situation of the patient/client. Each stage may vary in the proportional amount of time taken to pass through. In general, it should be borne in mind that the counsellor's aim is to use his or her own skills to develop the client's skills and learning to pass through each of the stages. The whole process can take minutes, days or weeks. One should also bear in mind that Egan encourages the novice counsellor not to apply the model too rigidly. He calls for flexibility to facilitate the helping process. He reminds us that human problems do not always lend themselves to this neat and clean set of sequences. Since human problems have many different components and complexities the counsellors may find themselves backtracking to earlier steps in the model before the client can move on in the process. This is consistent with a common view that effective learning in professional practice encourages the professional to develop personal models for action (Schon, 1987; Benner, 1984).

Stage I: Exploring the Present Scenario

Egan identifies the following steps in the development of Stage I. They are:

1. Helping clients to tell their stories. Here the counsellor and client are undertaking a search for the facts.
2. Identifying and challenging blind spots. Blind spots are elements of the problem situation that the client cannot see. The aim here is to explore alternative points of view and alternative interpretations of events.
3. The search for leverage. This is a consideration of the importance of the problem to the client or the priority that the problem has over other problems. It also involves clarifying the important elements of the problem.

Stage II: Developing a preferred scenario

The steps in this stage are:

1. Preferred-scenario possibilities. Here the client is encouraged to explore or imagine a better state of affairs. It explores the feasibility of change and the person potential for change. It generates options for change.
2. Creating viable agendas. This involves choosing from the better states of affairs those that are desirable and that make most sense. This is then transformed into an agenda or plan that has potential for fulfilment.
3. Making choices and commitments. The feasible outcomes or agenda that the client has generated is likely to be inspiring but sometimes elements may not be motivating enough to encourage action. Here the client and counsellor work toward examining the benefits of commitment to particular elements of the agenda.

Step III: Formulating strategies and plans

There are also three steps in this stage:
1. Brainstorming strategies for action. Once the agenda or feasible outcomes have secured some commitment then the possible options for action are explored.

2. Choosing the best strategies. Here there is a search for the actions that best fit the client's needs and lifestyle.
3. Turning strategies into a plan. This is essentially the drawing up of a step-by-step procedure for achieving the desired outcomes. It requires ordering and the inclusion of realistic time-frames.

This whole process requires the development of several skills that are required by the counsellor in order to develop skills in the client. The aim of the counselling process is to for both parties to share and develop their skill to arrive at a satisfactory outcome of that counselling process (Figure 7.3).

The skills that are required by the counsellor are worthy of review

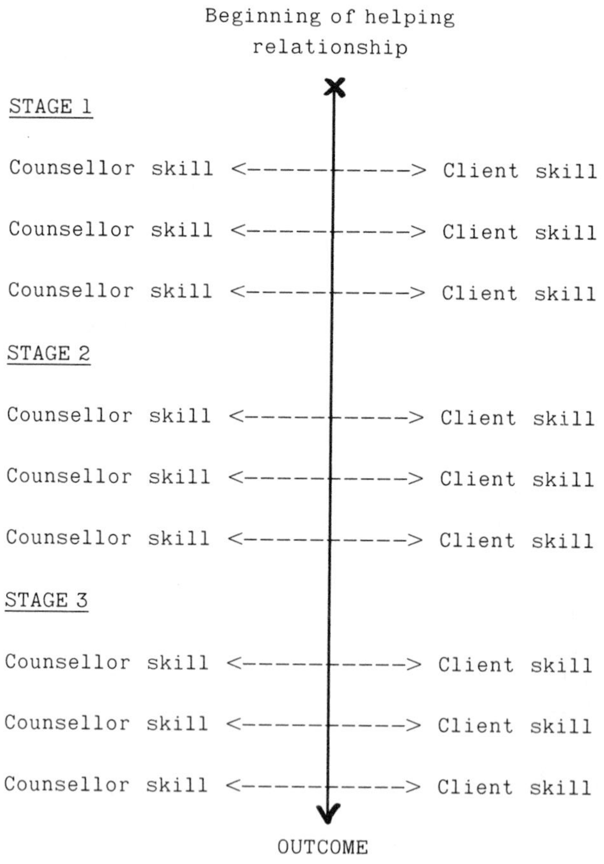

```
                    Beginning of helping
                       relationship
                            ✗
   STAGE 1                  |
                            |
   Counsellor skill <-------|------>  Client  skill
                            |
   Counsellor skill <-------|------>  Client  skill
                            |
   Counsellor skill <-------|------>  Client  skill
                            |
   STAGE 2                  |
                            |
   Counsellor skill <-------|------>  Client  skill
                            |
   Counsellor skill <-------|------>  Client  skill
                            |
   Counsellor skill <-------|------>  Client  skill
                            |
   STAGE 3                  |
                            |
   Counsellor skill <-------|------>  Client  skill
                            |
   Counsellor skill <-------|------>  Client  skill
                            |
   Counsellor skill <-------|------>  Client  skill
                            ▼
                         OUTCOME
```

Figure 7.3 Skill-sharing.

here and a summary is shown in the list following. Many items in the list of skills are derived from the work of Egan (1990) and are given in order of increasing probability of use as the process develops. Many will be appropriate to all stages of the model. The following list is a summary of counsellor skills.

1. Present scenario:
   (a) Attending.
   (b) Showing respect.
   (c) Genuineness.
   (d) Active listening.
   (e) Open questioning.
   (f) Dealing with resistance.
   (g) Coping with defence mechanisms.
   (h) Dealing with silence.
2. Preferred scenario:
   (a) Empathic understanding.
   (b) Challenging.
   (c) Self-disclosure.
   (d) Immediacy.
   (e) Eliciting new scenarios.
   (f) Stating personal goals.
   (g) Formulating personal objectives.
3. Formulating plans:
   (a) Balance-sheet analysis.
   (b) Decision-making.
   (c) Facilitating learning.
   (d) Sustaining action.
   (e) Referral.
   (f) Terminating the helping process.

As the counsellor uses his or her skills at each stage of the process, the skills of the client will also be brought in to play. Some skills the client will possess already and some will need to be developed by the counsellor. On some occasions, it may be prudent for the counsellor to compensate for any lack of skill in the client but the long-term aim should be client-empowerment by skill acquisition. In a truly sharing climate the counsellor will find that he or she is also developing as a person and learning. The client is providing stimulus for the skill development of the counsellor. Some of the client skills that may be developed are as follows:

1. Present scenario:
   (a) Attending.
   (b) Showing respect.
   (c) Genuineness.

  (d) Listening.
  (e) Ownership of the problem.
  (f) Describing thoughts.
  (g) Describing feelings.
  (h) Challenging.
  (i) Self-reflection.
  (j) Self-acceptance.
  (k) Dealing with silence.
2. Preferred scenario:
  (a) Identifying blind spots.
  (b) Self-disclosure.
  (c) Use of imagination.
  (d) Generation of options.
  (e) Giving and receiving strokes.
  (f) Imagination.
  (g) Creating new scenarios.
  (h) Stating personal goals.
3. Formulating plans:
  (a) Formulating objectives.
  (b) Balance-sheet analysis.
  (c) Decision-making.
  (d) Taking control of learning.
  (e) Sustaining action.

A REVIEW OF COUNSELLOR SKILLS

Attending

'The actively attending helper gives the client cues that he or she is present. These cues encourage the client to talk' (Egan 1975). For this skill, nurse counsellors aim to enter into the counselling process by devoting all their attention to the patient, both physically and psychologically. Nurses show that they are accepting the patients, recognizing his or her difficulty and are willing to spend time and energy on him or her. The skill of attending uses non-verbal signals in response to the verbal and non-verbal initiative taken by the patient/client.

  Some of the crucial non-verbal cues demonstrated by the counsellor are proximity, posture and orientation. The nurse must be spatially close enough to the patient to demonstrate 'psychological' closeness. It is not conducive to attending when the nurse is busy with some other task or positioned at the opposite corner of the room. Similarly, objects between the nurse and the patient, such as desks, tables or other people, can be restrictive. The counsellor must adopt an open orientation to the client facing his direction, most suitably seated at a right-angle. Face-to-face interaction is often construed as threatening. The nurse counsellor must judge the required orientation and closeness by being sensitive to the patient's non-verbal cues and even asking him or her where he or she would like to sit (or be positioned). It is also worth remembering that the level of eye contact is also important. When the nurse is standing over the seated or bed-bound patient it conveys an air of dominance – the person feels vulnerable (Figure 7.4). This is why the most skilled communicators bend their knees so that the face is at the same level as the face of the other person who they are communicating with – try this with children, patients in bed or students in the classroom, it facilitates communication and maximizes the feeling of equality. Some nurses naturally sit on the patient's bed and this is good so long as trust or permission has been secured as it can also be seen as an invasion of territory or an anxiety provoking situation. If the patient is bed-bound it is advisable to sit in a chair to talk to him or her. Sitting slouched in a chair (Figure 7.5) will not demonstrate attending, neither will resting apathetically on one knee.

Crossed arms and legs often indicate barriers to communication and open posture (Figure 7.6) is best adopted. Attending is shown by sitting upright and slightly forward in the direction of the person.

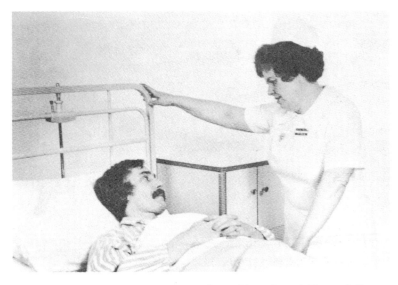

Figure 7.4 Towering over a patient confirms his vulnerability and the nurse's dominant attitude.

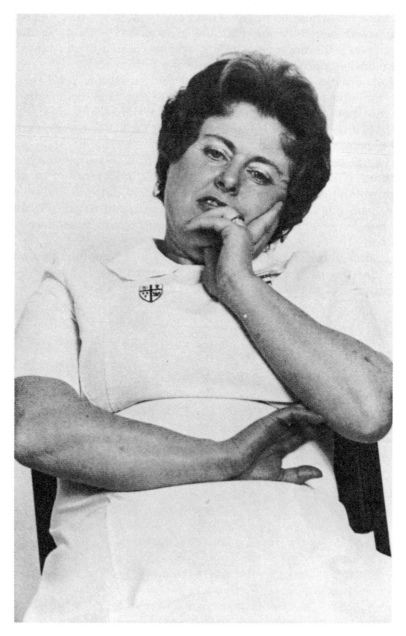

Figure 7.5 Is she really interested?

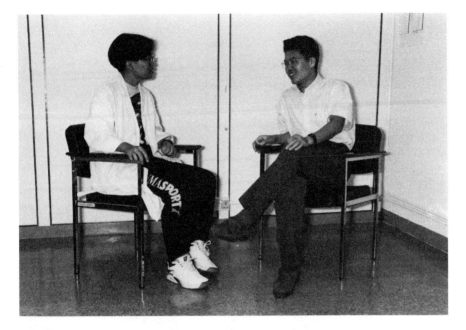

Figure 7.6 An open posture.

A final point on attending is eye contact and the direction of gaze. Quick looks at the clock, out of the window or at the intravenous infusion betray the fact that the nurse is not attending. Look at the person frequently to give feedback. Argyle and Dean have found that there is more gaze (looking in the direction of the other) when listening than when speaking. Speakers look up at the end of their utterances and at the beginning. It is at these times that they are checking to see if the other person is listening. It is also at these times that they are most prone to discouragement. Looking away at this point makes the speaker feel that they should stop. Interrupting at this point makes them stop. Other signs of attentiveness described by Argyle (1972) include head-nodding, reflective body posture (e.g. mirroring) and a slight tilt of the head. The need to use non-verbal skills is emphasized here because the nurse counsellor is best involved in 'passive listening' at the outset of the counselling process when attending is likely to engender trust.

Passive listening involves keeping the mouth closed and the ears open (Figure 7.7).

In conclusion it is worth remembering an important point made by Egan (1975): 'Don't focus on any one of the elements of attending so closely that attending itself becomes unnatural. . .'.

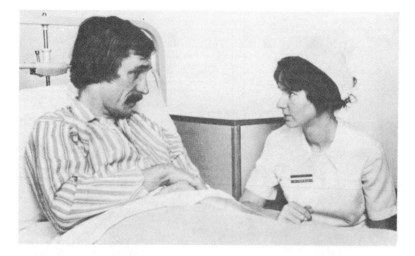

Figure 7.7 Attention-giving – looking in the direction of the other.

Showing Respect

The human need for respect has been said to be one of the strongest human needs (Egan, 1990). Egan says that showing respect is achieved by at least **doing no harm** to the person; this is also an old maxim of Florence Nightingale's. Doing the person no harm requires that the needs of the counsellor do not take precedence over the needs of the client especially where it is detrimental to the client. This can be seen as a form of exploitation. One of the forms of showing respect is to keep the client safe from counsellor exploitation by constantly reflecting and accepting one's own motives and needs as a counsellor. Another issue in showing respect is **treating the client as an individual**.

This is an important value for nurses. Another critical feature of respect is the **suspension of value judgements**. In showing respect one is consciously attempting to suspend personal judgements, opinions, attitude and feelings about the issues raised and working toward accepting the client's values, feelings and opinions. This is not easy to do at first but constant reflective practice can minimize our natural tendencies to judge others and allow our feeling to affect our caring responses to them. In order to maintain this skill of showing respect, two conditions should prevail:

1. Nurses should be aware of their own beliefs, values and prejudices, and be aware of and be able to accept that other people have different beliefs, values and habits. The skills of self-reflection and

self-acceptance are important but the skill of unconditionally accepting others for what they are is probably a more sophisticated ability.

2. Nurses also require some ability to control the expression or manifestations of their beliefs, values and prejudices, i.e. to curb their inclinations to express them, impose them or even mention them to the client. Those who are prone to adopting critical parent ego state should be most wary (see Chapter 4). This will also involve the management of non-verbal cues. Raised eyebrows, widened eyes, the dropped jaw, a sharp intake of breath, looking away and facial grimacing can all too easily indicate disapproval. Caring is about being on the same side as the person not about being opposed to him. The same is true of respect.

Carkhuff (1969) has described three features of showing respect. The first is that the counsellor communicates to the client – 'With me you are free to be who you are' – but that this is not wholly unconditional. The counsellor suspends judgement but does not reinforce or encourage client behaviour that may be harmful to the client or others.

The second feature is the ability of the counsellor to communicate that there are aspects of the client's situation that are worthy of help and understanding. The counsellor is positively responding to the client. Carkhuff says 'At a maximum, a depth of understanding on the part of the helper communicates his [or her] readiness and desire to be able to know the helpee more fully'.

The third of Carkhuff's means of showing respect seems at first to break with the non-judgmental approach. It involves reinforcing positive behaviours and withholding reinforcement of others. The important principle to adopt is that positive disapproval is not shown. Finally, Egan (1990) suggests other forms of showing respect: being available, communicating understanding, assuming the client's good will, being warm with reason, using the client's own resources and help with psychological pain are all elements of showing respect.

Genuineness

On genuineness Egan says of the counsellor:

> His [or her] offer of help cannot be phoney. He [or she] must be spontaneous, open. He [or she] can't hide behind the role of counsellor. He [or she] must be a human being to the human being before him [or her].
>
> *Egan, 1990*

Genuineness involves being open in both posture and attitude. The counsellor must be natural not false, be real not an actor. Many of the demands of the nurse's role can lead to attitudes that militate against genuineness in counselling situations. There are often compulsions to become over-procedural because of institutionalization or the stereotyped role of the nurse. When nurses consider that they are 'being paid to do this' or that it is 'what they are expected to do', then genuineness can be difficult to achieve. One must be genuinely concerned and want to help for this to be communicated to the patient/client. Carkhuff suggests two stages of genuineness. The first is 'minimization of maintaining a facade and playing the role'. He emphasizes the importance of the counsellor achieving accurate awareness of his or her own thoughts and behaviour in the counselling situation and adds: 'The helper will find that [he or] she is most effective when [he or] she concentrates upon understanding the helpee in relation to himself [herself] and his [her] own direction known to the helpee.'.

Egan (1990) suggests some further guidelines for communicating genuineness. They are:

- do not overemphasize the helping role;
- be spontaneous;
- avoid defensiveness;
- be consistent;
- work at becoming comfortable with the behaviour that helps the client.

Active listening

This is concerned with responding to the patient/client in a way that shows him or her that the nurse counsellor has listened and understood his or her point of view. It differs from passive listening in that it allows for the use of verbal responses by the counsellor. The verbal responses must only communicate the counsellor's understanding and should not add information that has originated from the counsellor. The focus of awareness must be on the patient's/client's life situation and should not be marred by the interpretations and speculations of the counsellor. This is also a useful principle for promoting patient-centredness in nursing generally. Three techniques have been described that can assist active listening; they are reflecting, paraphrasing and summarizing.

Reflecting

This is the act of merely repeating a word, pair of words or sentence exactly as it was said. It has the effect of underlining symbolically what the counsellor considers to be a crucial point. It may indicate that the listener is attuned to the issues that the client finds important. It may also serve to encourage the client to expand on that point. An example of this is shown in the following dialogue, where P represents the patient and N the nurse.

P: 'I can't seem to get used to this bag, I don't like it. . .Why did this have to happen to me? (Pause) It's so awkward, you'd think they would invent something better. Its so smelly!' (Pause).

N: 'Smelly?'

P: 'Yes, you can see it on people's faces, the visitors and the other patients, even the nurses. I even get sick of it myself. I've got some special discs to put in but I don't know how I'm going to cope at home, parties and such like, I'll never be able to go to the golf club.'

N: 'You'll never be able to go to the golf club?'

P: 'No, I think I'll have to give that up because of this pong.'

Two points should be borne in mind when using this reflective response. One is that this response should not be overused or sound forced. Let the repetition come naturally even if you add the odd extra word. Be resilient. One can imagine the effect of the nurse's overzealous use of reflecting (Figure 7.8).

Paraphrasing

This is a skill that involves the activity of putting the client's statement, thoughts or feelings into one's own words. By choosing different words one can crystallize the ideas and feelings of the client. This may achieve two things. The first is that the counsellor demonstrates his or her degree of understanding of what the client has said, particularly the deeper meaning. The second effect is that of the 'sounding board' effect. The counsellor in this situation acts as a mirror to reflect the client's comments, allowing the client to experience the effect of his or her comments on the counsellor and so receive some feedback on the presentation of his or her opinions and self. In the example of paraphrasing below, the nurse is responding to a 45-year-old soldier who has had to have an above-knee amputation of his left leg.

P: 'Something keeps nagging away at the back of my mind. I know its childish to make such a big thing about losing a leg. It's a sorry state if a man can't take such things in his stride, particularly at my time of life. . . but it keeps me awake at night.'

N: 'Are you saying that you feel that your reaction to the loss of your leg is some sort of weakness?'

P: 'Yeh, I'd never have thought that I could be like this. . .'.

Sometimes the use of similes and metaphors during paraphrasing can bring a unique dimension to this response. Nevertheless, the

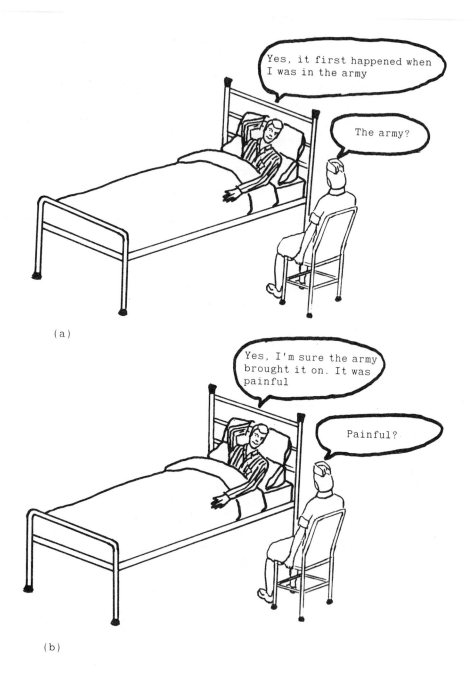

(a)

(b)

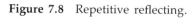

Figure 7.8 Repetitive reflecting.

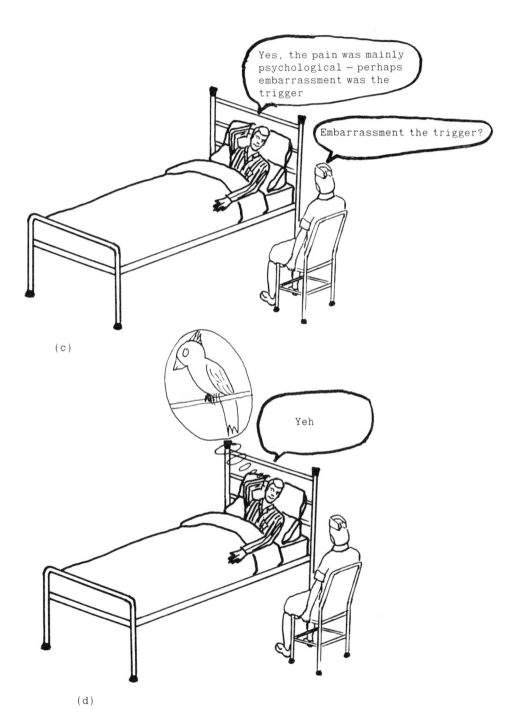

(c)

(d)

counsellor should remember not to use sayings that the person may not be familiar with.

Summarizing

This embodies the activity of: (i) picking out the main points from a fairly large amount of dialogue or from a long protracted disclosure; (ii) condensing these points into a short phrase; (iii) using the client's words where possible; and (iv) ensuring that the content, as well as expressed feelings are included in the points chosen. One would then allow the client time to respond to this summary, adding to it or altering some of the main points mentioned. Summarizing helps both counsellor and client to focus on the main issues and to begin to assess the relative importance of the points made. Let us look at an example of a nurse's summarizing response to a lucid elderly lady who has been told by the doctor that she can go home in a few days time.

   P: 'I'm not looking forward to going out you know. I've got so many places to go, I don't know what to do. . .'.

   N: 'Really!'

   P: 'My son said that he would have me. I could stay in the spare room, which would become mine of course. But Enid, my daughter-in-law, is so house proud she said I can't take Jimmy (the cat) and I would have to leave my old jugs, ornaments and knickknacks like my lavender bag, for the house clearers to sell. Anyway I think she only wants to get her hands on my pension. Then there's my friend Alice, she wants me to live with her, but she's *** and I've heard she goes a bit funny at night, wandering you know. . .'.

   N: 'Mmm. . .'

   P: 'I can't stay in my house because you never know what's going to happen to you or if anybody's going to know. But I do love my little house, I've been there 45 years, you know. Me and Jack, God bless him, moved there just after he came back from France out of the army. . .'

   N: 'Yeh?'

   P: 'And on top of all that, the social worker said that I can have an old person's flat, but you're still on your own then, aren't you?'

   N: 'So you don't know whether to go home, or to stay with your son, to stay with Alice or take an old person's flat, and this is getting you really confused?'

   P: 'Well you see I don't want to upset anyone. They've all been very kind.'

Hays and Larson (1963) have suggested the following additional opening comments when summarizing:

- 'Have I got this straight?'.
- 'You've said that. . .'.
- 'During the past hour you and I have discussed. . .'.

Others may include:

- 'Now let's see what I think you have said';
- 'It seems that what you are trying to say is that';
- 'It appears that you are telling me that. . .'.

It should always be borne in mind that interjections such as reflecting, paraphrasing and summarizing can direct the client's commentary in two ways. The first is by signposting important points. As described before, this aspect may be put to good use; however, overuse may cause the discussion to follow the counsellor's interests rather than the expressive needs of the patients. In addition interjections by the counsellor may interrupt the client's train of thought if used inappropriately. These responses should be used at pauses in conversation when it is obvious that the client is not going to pursue another point. They should definitely be used between sentences or just as the person draws breath to begin again. It must be emphasized that it is the counsellor's aim to communicate understanding and empathy not to demonstrate how well he or she can reflect or paraphrase. The tendency to do this may be counteracted if the counsellor develops what Egan has called the ability of the counsellor to listen to himself or herself during the counselling interview itself.

Open Questioning

Introducing open or free-answer questions gives freedom of choice to the client to answer in whatever way he or she wishes. These types of question allow spontaneity and most usefully allow clients to share opinions, values, beliefs and feelings. It has also been suggested (Hargie *et al.*, 1981) that they allow the respondent a greater degree of control over the interaction. For these reasons, open questions are particularly helpful in helping the client to explore present and preferred scenarios. If one wants to ensure that open questions are asked, it is advisable to start with the 'How', 'What' or 'In what way' and avoid beginnings that use the word 'Why?. It is not always easy to formulate open questions and practice will improve this ability. Look below at the following nurse's questions in closed and open form.

Closed	Open
1. Do you think your relatives don't come because they have more important things to do?	What do you think stops your relatives coming to see you?

| 2. Will you be able to cope back home? | In what way do you think things will be different when you go back home? |

An alternative way of eliciting open responses is by phrases that are not questions at all but have the same effect. Phrases such as the following are actually instructions but they do not appear this way in a climate of trust an caring:

- 'Explain to me about your relatives.'
- 'Tell me more about how you think things will be when you get back home.'
- 'I'm interested to know more about. . .'.
- 'Tell me about yourself.'

During the exploration of present scenarios eliciting open response is particularly effective. Probing and leading questions are generally inappropriate until trust has genuinely been established. A type of open question called the affective question has been described by Hargie *et al.* (1981). These questions refer directly to emotions, attitudes and feelings. Examples of such questions may be: 'How do you feel about going for the gastroscopy tomorrow?'; 'What are your feelings now?'; 'This must have hurt you, can you tell me more about it?'. Remember that the nurse counsellor's aim is to encourage the person to tell the story about the present scenario or to imagine a preferred scenario.

Coping with resistance

Resistance is the phenomenon in which a person mobilizes his or her resources or feelings against the helper. It is negative and can be destructive to the relationship and the counsellor personally. It will often thwart the aims of counselling and cause frustration in the over-zealous counsellor.

The crucial issue about resistance is to recognize it as soon as possible. Sim (1969) suggests that resistance may be demonstrated in the client by periods of silence, rudeness, irrelevant comment or irreverent remarks. This may be a serious indication of a lack of trust in the counsellor or that the client has spotted a lack of respect or genuineness. It is most important to backtrack at this stage and make one's primary aim the building of trust rather than the development of the present of preferred scenarios. Immediacy, by talking about the cause of the client's 'unhappiness' can help if it appears that the counselling relationship is going to come to a halt. This action may prove to be a turning point in the development of the relationship. It is possible that the resistant response is a part of the client's problem. Freud (1914) suggests that resistance should be 'worked through' and overcome. The greatest problem for the counsellor in this situation is his or her own feelings and frustration. It is easy to give up on the person as an 'impossible case'. Resistance does not indicate a dislike for the counsellor as a person and once it is seen as an area that the client needs help with and not as an expression of ungratefulness, resistance can be overcome by building on trust and showing acceptance and genuineness.

Coping with Defence Mechanisms

There are many things that clients do that can be attributed to defence mechanisms. In Freudian psychology (1901), these are ego defence mechanisms or psychological mechanisms that protect our self-image. These responses are subconscious and have a very important function. They are normal **not** abnormal responses. The function of a defence mechanism is to protect people from the emotional agony of having to accept facts about themselves that they find intolerable. Were it not for defence mechanisms, most individuals would suffer such anxiety from emotional conflict that they would find it difficult to live a satisfactory or productive life. Mental illness would undoubtedly ensue. Removing the protection of ego defence often causes conflict and emotional pain. The affected person will see those who pierce his or her defence as callous and to some extent they are. Those in intimate helping relationships with others have a duty to preserve these defences and should only confront the person with them in a tentative careful fashion. Only a highly skilled professional counsellor should confront a person with his or her defence mechanisms.

Recognition of defence mechanisms is crucial to the process of counselling. In order to achieve this the nurse counsellor must know how the different types of ego defence manifest themselves.

The possible ego defence mechanisms are as follows:

1. Rationalization is justifying an action, thought or attitude so that it appears reasonable when otherwise it would appear irrational, e.g. 'I knew I wouldn't pass my examination, I never did like the subject.'
2. Reaction formation is a defence against unacceptable wishes or urges that involves the person saying or doing things that are totally the opposite of the unacceptable wishes.
3. Repression is the active process of forgetting things that are too painful to contemplate.
4. Projection is highlighting one's own ideas, behaviours, mistakes or faults to another person in the hope that they will not be attributed to oneself.
5. Denial is refusing to accept the existence of a personal attribute.

Others include suppression, regression, displacement, dissociation, sublimation, conversion and fantasy. The reader is advised to look to psychology texts or dictionaries for a fuller understanding of these concepts.

Dealing with Silence

Silence often occurs during counselling and similar situations. It can be extremely uncomfortable for the persons involved probably because we have learned that silence is a cue to turn-taking during conversation. Habits that we develop in everyday social conversation are often carried over into situations that do not require vocal communication. The uncomfortable and even tension-producing effects of silence can be both an advantage and a disadvantage. Silence can be put to good use by the counsellor in that it can encourage the client to talk. This will require some patience. Silence becomes a problem, however, where the counsellor has no patience and attempts to continue the flow of dialogue from the client by asking questions or phrases for active listening. Observation of the client's non-verbal cues is crucial if the counsellor is to decide whether the silence is productive for the client or not. Silence can be a resting period for both participants in the counselling process, it may be a period of crucial reflection for either of them. The understanding and acceptance of new ideas or feelings that cause initial conflict often require a period of silence. When a person needs to formulate his or her thoughts, words and sentences they are often silent for quite long periods. Some people are more reflective than others. Silence can also be a period to test out the trust that exists between two people. Very often we are quite happy in silence with the people we love or trust. When we feel comfortable about not having to talk, there is a certain trust in the other person. As a general strategy, it is as well for the nurse counsellor to observe and wait for some time before speaking. The patient/client will let him or her know by non-verbal means if he or she wants the counsellor to say something or will begin talking when he or she is ready. If the counsellor is uncertain after a long period of silence it is sometimes appropriate to ask some closed questions to check out the situation such as: 'Are you sorting out your thoughts?'; 'Are you thinking about what we have just said?': 'Is this a time to rest and collect our thoughts?'.

Within this advice it is worth remembering that there are also personality differences in the way in which each of us uses silence. Lewis (1973) described four types of personality that adopt silence for different reasons. In their observations during silent periods it is as well for nurses to consider some of these personality differences. The **taciturn** person is one who is silent because he or she is habitually uncommunicative. The **reserved** person causes silences by being

withdrawn in speech and self-restrained in manner. Lewis describes
reticence as a disinclination or an embarrassment to disclose feelings
or personal information. The final form of silence may be exemplified
by the **secretive** person, who conceals or is evasive because of the
habit of being suspicious. Remember that these responses do not
mean that the client has any less value as a human being. Indeed,
many nurse counsellors need to control these tendencies in themselves.

Silence does not necessarily indicate reluctance, dislike, uncoopera-
tiveness or aggression, yet the feeling that it does is the nurse
counsellor's greatest enemy. Baker (1955) has described two types of
silence: (i) positive, which characterizes intimacy and harmony; and
(ii) negative, which points to animosity and hostility. It will be
necessary for the nurse to identify the type of silence in order to deal
with it. Positive silence is a benefit allowing the client and counsellor
to become more aware of their inner selves and each other. It is a sign
of trust when silence can take place without the participants feeling
pressurized. Negative silence may need to be dealt with by tolerance,
checking and immediacy.

Empathic Understanding

Egan (1975) describes this skill as the communication of an understanding of the client by the counsellor that goes beyond the words
used to the implications or latent meaning of what has been said. It
tries to precipitate implied feelings or thoughts. Here the nurse
counsellor is making tentative guesses and suggestions about ideas
and feelings that the client may be unaware of and perhaps unable to
accept. Egan says that the helper begins to make connections between
seemingly isolated statements made by the client. The sub-skill of
summarizing will be of value here, but Egan makes the important
point that nothing must be added by the counsellor, the focus must
remain with the client and the counsellor should not add material of
his or her own invention. This is why he uses the word 'accurate' in
his description of this skill. It must fix precisely on the client's view of
the world and his or her self-understanding.

Empathy means the ability to appreciate another person's thoughts
and feelings from his or her point of view. It is putting yourself 'in
another person's shoes'. It differs from sympathy in that sympathy
involves sharing another person's feelings, being affected in a similar
way by them. Empathy, being somewhat more objective, seems to be
more appropriate to nursing. This does not, however, mean that the
nurse should have no feelings for the other person.

It has been known for nurses to be advised by their colleagues that
they should not get involved with the patient. Even that we should

remain emotionally detached. This amounts to saying that we should be non-human and not care for the patient. It is interesting that many nurses and scholars use the phrase 'nursing care' as a euphemism for nursing work. It is a traditional cliché. Care is not a practical word it is an emotive word and betrays the fact that nursing is an emotional as well as an objective pursuit. Empathy should not be confused with sympathy, which can be said to indicate a situation in which the patient's/client's emotions are reinforced and shared by the nurse counsellor in an unhelpful way, without the development of mutual understanding. Sympathy condones, often unreservedly, the feeling state of the client and the main purpose is to demonstrate kindness or emotional compatibility. Empathy can be considered to be a state of affairs in which the nurse counsellor has an understanding of the patient's/client's situations and adequately reflects this understanding to him or her. It can also be said that an ability to be empathetic it is necessary to develop an ability to be less self-focused. Being overly concerned with oneself and one's self-presentation is a common and somewhat human trait. In order to be empathetic is useful to be aware of our self-concern. This is why it is useful for the counsellor to have a degree of self-awareness that inspires personal confidence. During the skill of accurate empathy, the boundaries of the client self-knowledge are stretched and thus there is the possibility of extending the counsellor's empathic understanding. Carkhuff describes this admirably when he says: 'It is as if the helper, having successfully formulated the helpee's world, stands up in it and stretches out his or her arms and legs to reach its corners and crevices'. Advanced accurate empathy may be achieved in several ways by the nurse counsellor:

1. By identifying themes i.e. by tentatively suggesting thoughts or trends that run like continuous threads through the previous conversations. For example, one may say, 'This idea of loneliness seems to have been mentioned several times; is this a major concern?'.

2. Helping the client to come to the ultimate conclusions of what has been said, i.e. encouraging him or her to foresee what would be most likely to happen, e.g. 'What do you think would happen if you can not persuade John to go to school?'.

3. By pointing to possible bridges or links between seemingly unrelated issues, facts or feelings, e.g. 'Do you see any way in which your comment about disliking authority is linked to your relationship with Sister Blewitt?'.

4. Stating clearly things that the client may have said in vague, disjointed or confused terms, for example:

   P: I'm not sure about this operation. It seems. . .well, silly to have it, but its for my own sake, so they say. . . .But I'm not convinced. . . . It doesn't look as if I have any alternative, although I suppose we all have the right to make up our own minds.

N: It seems as though you are saying that you do not want to have the operation? **or** I can sense that you feel pressurized into having the operation.

Egan (1990) gives some practical advice in the form of what to do and what not to do. Do:

- give yourself time to think;
- use short responses;
- gear your response to the client but be yourself.

Do not (mainly consists of poor responses):

- give no response at all;
- ask inappropriate questions;
- utter clichés;
- offer an interpretation;
- give advice;
- pretend to understand;
- reply in parrot fashion;
- offer sympathy or agreement.

From this form of empathy it is hoped that the acquired understanding indicates problems worthy of solution. Carkhuff, in his third stage of empathy, stresses the importance of turning to action in problem-solving.

Challenging

This is most appropriate to the second step of Stage 1 of Egan's model, which is the identification of blind spots. In one way, this is more provocative than many of the strategies outlined above.

Challenging is concerned with the elimination of blind spots and the opening up of new perspectives. When the nurse counsellor identifies a perspective that the patient/client has obviously not identified then the process of challenging is about offering this alternative viewpoint as a stimulus for further consideration. It is an interesting feature of counselling that many individuals actually need the help of a counsellor simply because they cannot see or do not want to accept the 'obvious'. It is useful to remember that challenging should be a carefully thought out, positive and caring response. Egan relates six types of client response that can be challenged.

1. Failure to own problems.
2. Failure to define problems in solvable terms.
3. Faulty interpretations of critical experiences, behaviours and feelings.
4. Evasions, distortions and game-playing.
5. Failure to identify or understand the consequences of behaviour.
6. Hesitancy or unwillingness to act on new perspectives.

Self-disclosure

Self-disclosure is the act of sharing personal experience with the client. The nurse counsellor briefly describes something that has happened to him or her or some feeling he or she has experienced in the hope that it will throw some new light on the patient's/client's problem. It also has two other possible effects. Self-disclosure may demonstrate to the client the fact that the counsellor identifies with his or her problem. The counsellor understands the client's experience because he or she has been affected by similar events. In addition, self-disclosure demonstrates the counsellor's trust in the client by disclosing hitherto private information. If the client discloses private thoughts or information in a climate of trust, then it seems appropriate that the counsellor can do the same in this climate of mutual trust. This will help to develop the relationship as well as the counselling process.

Self-disclosure should be of benefit to the client. The counsellor should be wary that self-disclosure does not bring about a role reversal, where the counsellor is eliciting help and the client is becoming the helper. It is important not to take the focus away from the client's concerns by placing the burden of the counsellor's problems on the client. Examples of some self-disclosing comments are:

1. 'Yes, I can understand how important the pain is to you. When I have pain and nobody takes any notice, I get frustrated and it seems to get worse. Is this the way you feel or does it affect you differently?'
2. 'I was divorced myself some years ago and I also found it strange that I lost what I thought were good friends because they were shocked.'

Immediacy

Egan describes this as 'you/me' talk. It actually involves describing what is going on, here and now, between the counsellor and client. It is a way of standing outside of the issues to look at the relationship or the counselling process. It removes the focus from the issues that are of concern to the client to reflections on how both parties are behaving toward each other, how they respond to each other and how they are coping with the interaction. Immediacy, as a skill, involves frank, open and direct reference to what is going on at the moment. Inskipp *et al.* (1978) suggest the following structure for immediacy comments: (i) I; (ii) then a feeling; (iii) then a reason. For example, 'I feel as though you do not really want to tell me the real story. I think I am doing something to put you off. Is this true?'.

Some difficulties in communicating may point to the fact that the counsellor and the client have achieved no rapport. It may be that the client does not want to share problems or does not want the help offered. Immediacy may therefore be used in such instances and where resistance occurs. Immediacy is a powerful source of feedback about the relationship and by defining the situation, the client and counsellor may come to appreciate behaviour that one is displaying and which may be misunderstood by the other. Carkhuff points to two stages of immediacy. The first is preparatory and takes the form of tentative hints about how the client is relating to the counsellor. For example, 'You seem to notice something about me that is making it difficult for you to talk. Am I right? Can you describe it?'. The second stage of immediacy can then move toward 'I/feeling/reason' comments. Egan (1990) has refined the concept of immediacy and distinguishes between three types of immediacy:

1. Self-involving statements, which convey the counsellor's positive personal opinions about progress that the client is making, e.g. 'I am really flattered that you talk to me more about your feelings compared to when we first met'.
2. Relationship immediacy, which enables the counsellor to give feedback about his or her perceptions of the nature of the relationship with the client. 'We seem to get on OK even though I have sometimes misunderstood you. You never seem to get angry with me when I don't understand you. I wonder why you say you easily become angry with your husband when he doesn't understand you?'.
3. Here-and-now immediacy, which encourages the counsellor, and sometimes the client, to stand back and look at a particular incident that is causing problems in the interaction between them both: 'Suddenly I feel really awkward when I ask you a question. Am I doing something wrong?'.

Immediacy should help the client to understand more about himself or herself and his or her relationship with the counsellor. It may be of use in any stage of the counselling process.

Eliciting New Scenarios

Egan describes several strategies that can be adopted when helping others to create new and better scenarios. They are:

1. Asking future-oriented questions, or trying to frame questions in ways that ask about how things could be, how things would be better and how things could be different to the way they are now.
2. Helping clients find models, which means helping clients to identify people who they respect and exploring how these people would deal with the issues.
3. Reviewing better times, by looking at instances in the past where issues were resolved satisfactorily or conditions were more favourable.
4. Helping clients get involved in new experiences, and discovering different outlooks on life. Changes in leisure activities, occupation, lifestyle, routines, location, friends or partners may bring fresh perspectives and even a new appreciation of these aspects of the present scenario.
5. Using writing approaches, this is a method of clarifying thoughts and communicating with oneself in an almost objective way. The creative element of writing poetry, short stories or letters can enable the development of imagination concerning a particular scenario.
6. Using fantasy, this a powerful way of achieving and developing imagination. Some people find it easier to fantasize than others, and one of the inhibitions to fantasizing is that it is not bound by reality and can seem to be ridiculous at times. When developing this skill it is important for the counsellor to be accepting and tolerant of another person's outlandish ideas.

Stating Personal Goals

Here the nurse counsellor is encouraging the client to develop skills in selecting particular outcomes that are feasible. A useful way of doing this is to encourage the client to brainstorm. This involves writing down anything at all, words or phrases that indicate things that he or she thinks will help. It is unnecessary to discuss the list in full but it may be necessary for the nurse counsellor and client to clarify some of the points made. This, however, should not be overdone. The next task for the client can now be to arrange this list of actions or requirements in order of importance. The points that the client sees as most useful should be placed at the top of the list, the second most important next and so on down the list. In this way a hierarchy of needs can be identified. A variation on this theme can be for the nurse to draw up a list of suggestions as well, in the belief that 'two heads are better than one'. This can also be an ideal opportunity for 'challenging', a skill described earlier in this section. The client could also be encouraged to consult with others about possible courses of action, particularly those who may be affected by the decision. All of these options are suggested to enhance the generation of a varied list of options.

It is important during this brainstorming activity that the counsellor does not comment on the ideas that the client generates. Passing value-judgements generally inhibits the generation of ideas and the purpose of brainstorming is to create as many options as possible.

Formulating personal objectives/target outcomes

This involves taking up the woolly or vague proposals for action and stating them in precise objective terms. Objectives should state the goal in terms of the desired outcome, situation or conditions that will indicate that the objective has been achieved. The objective should have built-in criterion or indicators that enable the client and others to recognize that the objective has been achieved. It is also useful if the client expresses the objective in his or her own words. An example might be: 'I would like to be able to forget about my stoma when I am at a party and at work with my workmates, to behave normally and not feel embarrassed'.

Another important element of an objective/outcome statement is that it should specify the conditions in which the persons should demonstrate the successful behaviour. For example, 'at a dinner party' or 'while with workmates', demonstrates attempts to specify the real-life conditions that should exist when demonstrating the successful behaviour.

Sometimes personal objectives can be very demanding and it may be necessary to break each one up into several achievable intermediate objectives. The counsellor should assist the client to identify a sequence of steps toward the final outcome that are ordered in terms of level of difficulty. An example relating to the above example for the stoma patient may look as follows:

1. An outcome concerned with being happy and willing to go out of the house to go to work.
2. An outcome concerned with staying in a room with a person for a short period of time without being self-conscious.
3. An outcome concerned with staying in close proximity to a friend or colleague for a long period of time.
4. An outcome concerned with staying in a crowded room for a long period of time.

It is not always necessary to be this detailed in breaking up outcomes and the overall principle of identifying outcomes with a reasonable prospect of success should be observed.

Balance-sheet Analysis

This is a development of Egan's force-field analysis (1975). It is an aid to decision-making that can be used by counsellors to help clients to identify gains and losses as well as the acceptability of these gains and losses to the individual, significant others and the social setting. In essence the client is assisted to complete a *pro forma* balance sheet recommended by Egan as shown in Figure 7.9.

The balance sheet should be completed by the client in his or her own words without any value judgement being forwarded by the counsellor. Perhaps the balance sheet will need to be modified several times as the counsellor and the client spend time sharing their thoughts on the contents of the balance sheet.

It is of interest that procedures such as this are also useful to the nurse in all of his or her 'partnership' activities with the patient. It is a useful means of negotiating supportive or remedial nursing care with the patient during the process of care planning. This is a process of problem-solving.

Decision-making

The process of decision-making differs from problem-solving in that it requires the selection of one option from several generated options. Stating personal goals, formulating personal objectives and balance-sheet analysis are all aids to decision-making. Decision-making requires some commitment to one option and the rejection of others. It often involves taking a risk. The chosen option may not turn out as good as another option. Sometimes people cannot make a decision because they are too cautious about taking a risk. Some people are too spontaneous and make quick decisions and, in these situations, the quality of these decisions can be poor. The counsellor will need to facilitate decision-making in both of these situations by using many of the skills outlined previously. It is important in the development of decision-making in others to encourage them to make decisions and to be decisive. In this case, practice makes perfect. Some people may not have sufficient experience of making decisions for themselves because significant other people in their lives have always made decisions for them. Occasionally, such people may make demands on the counsellor by displaying helpless behaviour. Sometimes the client will ask the counsellor what to do and, on other occasions it may be quite subtle, inducing the novice counsellor to give advice before realizing that he

If I choose this course of action:		
The self		
Gains for self:	Acceptable to me because:	Not acceptable to me because:
Losses for self:	Acceptable to me because:	Not acceptable to me because:
Significant others		
Gains for significant others:	Acceptable to me because:	Not acceptable to me because:
Losses for significant others:	Acceptable to me because:	Not acceptable to me because:
Social setting		
Gains for social setting:	Acceptable to me because:	Not acceptable to me because:
Losses for social setting:	Acceptable to me because:	Not acceptable to me because:

Figure 7.9 Balance sheet analysis (Egan, 1990).

or she has done so. Gelatt (1962) proposed a conceptual frame of reference for counselling that can help us to understand the thought processes that the client may be engaged in when making decisions (Figure 7.10).

The process begins with a clear understanding of the purpose or objective. The person then considers the data or information that he or

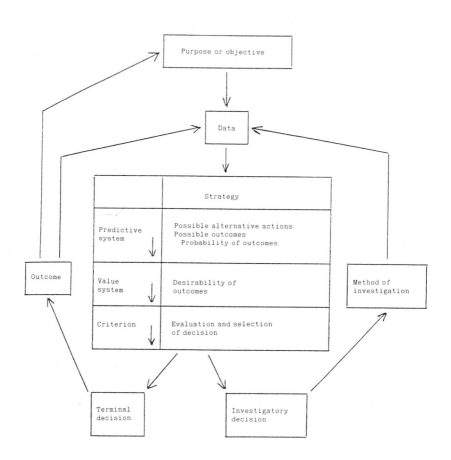

Figure 7.10 Gelatt's conceptual frame of reference for counselling.

she possesses about the problem. He or she then moves through a strategy system whereby he or she considers the feasibility of outcomes in a prediction system, the desirability of outcomes in a value system and finally he or she evaluates and selects an option in a criterion system. This model is synonymous with Egan's approach.

A useful element of Gelatt's model is that it provides for the possibility of making investigatory decisions. It also encourages us to accept that decision-making is a cyclical and not a linear process. The patient/client can still retrieve the situation where the decision seems to be ineffective and can even test out decisions before making a final commitment to them. It has been argued that most decision-making is of the risky type (Kozielecki, 1981). One of the critical skills of decision-making can, therefore, be said to be the ability to take risks. In the context of counselling, this is very important to remember because the trust and confidence that is developed in counselling is clearly beneficial in the pursuit of client decision-making. It is also advisable for the would-be nurse counsellor to engage in a little self-reflection on the subject of his or her own decision-making ability given that it is probably a benefit for the counsellor to be reasonably decisive without making decisions for the client.

Facilitating Learning

On some occasions, it may be useful for the client to learn different ways of responding or behaving. In addition, Egan suggests that the counsellor needs to 'help clients acquire the skills they need to act'. The skills outlined in this book can all be acquired by the client as well as the nurse counsellor.

The nurse can facilitate his learning in several ways. The description here will be brief because the facilitation of learning is discussed in greater depth later in this book.

Some of the following methods may be used to facilitate the client's learning:

- modelling;
- desensitization;
- imitation;
- relaxation;
- identification;
- information-giving;
- demonstration;
- assertiveness training;
- role-simulation.

For most of the methods of learning, the principle of feedback is significant. It is important for the counsellor to remember the following guidelines adapted from the work of Weinhold and Elliott (1979):

1. Give feedback about personal behaviour rather than about the person.
2. Make feedback specific and refer it to the person's present behaviour as it occurs.
3. Offer feedback that is helpful to the client and which is seen as helpful by him or her.
4. Do not make interpretations, give advice or ascribe motives.

Referral

Referral should not be seen by the nurse as a failing, for it is often the most sensible help that can be given to the client in helping towards action. The limitations of the nurse counsellor as a person and as a professional must be acknowledged and it is probable that others will have skills or experience that the nurse does not possess but which may be of enormous benefit to the patient/client. Clinebell (1966) points to several reasons for referral. The following list is influenced by his work:

1. The client can be helped more effectively by another.
2. The client does not respond to the counsellor's offers of help (e.g. shows resistance).
3. The client's needs take up too much of the would-be counsellor's time.
4. The client's needs are best met by established organizations (e.g. Alcoholics Anonymous).
5. The client has serious financial problems.
6. The client needs medical advice or specialist treatment.
7. The client seems to be suffering a mental illness or needs intensive psychotherapy.
8. The counsellor is doubtful about the nature of the client's problem.
9. The client is severely depressed or suicidal.
10. The counsellor has a dislike for the client and cannot overcome it.
11. The client's conflicts are of a religious nature and require religious support.

Referral from the nurse counsellor will often involve other members of the hospital and community health care team. The most obvious referrals will be to doctors, social workers, senior nurses, clinical nurse specialists, professions allied to medicine, the hospital chaplain, patients' organizations, marriage guidance counsellors and other specialist counsellors. Professional counsellors exist who specialize in helping with bereavement (e.g. Cruise), catastrophe, sexual problems, rape, child abuse and AIDS to name a few of the most common. Patients' organizations that are concerned with mental illness, mental handicap, epilepsy, mastectomy, stoma and diabetes provide sufficient evidence that many patients' organizations exist and that the effective nurse counsellor should always consider their existence if the patient needs specialized counselling help. Most of these organizations offer counsellors who have experience the same problems as the patient and who will visit to give a range of help and support to the patient/client.

A Dilemma of Confidentiality

The client's response to a suggestion for referral will either meet with approval or resistance from the client. The client's wishes must be respected. There are times, however, when the reason for considering referral is because the client is likely to do himself (or herself) or someone else some harm. Suicidal or violent thoughts provide two such examples. Even where referral is not being considered situations occur where the client may be harmed if action is not taken. There are times during counselling when it becomes appropriate to talk about confidentiality. One must always guarantee that what the client says will go no further unless he or she gives permission for a named other person to be told the personal information that has been shared with the counsellor. The client should know that he or she will be told before the counsellor shares this information and that his or her expressed permission will be sought. It is also useful to clarify precisely what will be said to the other person. The counsellor must stick to this agreement. The point of this whole exercise is to conserve the client's trust.

On very rare occasions, the client may not give permission for the counsellor to disclose information to another person. Some nurse counsellors have a dilemma here and have been known to value the ethic of confidentiality above the safety of the person. Clients should be helped to understand that the counsellor's role as a nurse and a caring human being cannot be compromised by an expectation to keep information secret at any price. Where a client does not agree to the disclosure of information such as 'I am thinking of killing myself tonight', then the nurse counsellor must risk the trust in the counsellor–client relationship. The nurse must tell the client that she is going to inform a named person about particular statements that the client has made, that she considers it necessary to save the client from serious harm and the reasons why she must do this. It should be explained to the client that the break in confidentiality will still remain restricted information. This does not mean that all the details of the client's disclosures should be given to others, only those that are essential. It is still possible to maintain confidentiality with respect to all other issues that have been shared in the counselling sessions that are personal, private and irrelevant to the perceived danger. One break in confidentiality does not mean that the client's private life can become an open book. Similarly, this option to disclose information against the client's wishes should not be taken lightly. It should not be perceived as an opt-out clause when the counsellor finds the counselling process too demanding. Breaking confidentiality is for the benefit of the client not the counsellor.

Terminating the Helping Process

It may seem strange to suggest that this is a skill but it is an acquired ability and something that some nurses may find hard to achieve. There are two occasions when this will occur, firstly at the end of a session. Many counselling relationships occur in a series of contacts or sessions separated in time periods of hours, days or weeks. So the nurse counsellor must find a way to end a session. The other time when the process must be brought to an end is when the client has come to a resolution of his conflict or problem. In essence, the helping process must come to an end when the client does not need help any more. The principles of set closure as outlined in the chapters on communication skills and interviewing are relevant to this situation. It is important to help the client to understand the time period that is available for counselling, to summarize what has happened in the session and to plan for the next meeting. When it is not necessary to arrange for another meeting then this should be understood clearly by both parties and follow a natural process of mutual agreement. Sometimes this will result in the termination of a caring relationship that may at times be quite mutually satisfying for both parties. It can be expected that the nurse counsellor and the patient/client can feel a sense of loss when the relationship comes to an end. This should not be ignored. The nurse should help the client to prepare for feelings of loss, if they exist, and find ways to help the client to cope. The nurse may also need the same sort of support from a colleague or senior counsellor.

SOME CONSIDERATIONS FOR NURSE COUNSELLING

After reading the literature on counselling one is usually led to assume that clients can communicate reasonably effectively with the counsellor. There are times, however, when it is difficult to counsel because the client is unable to articulate as well as the counsellor. It can be something of a problem for patients to understand the 'professional class' language of well-educated practitioners. Words such as: share, emotion, relationship or issue, may be considered unusual vocabulary for persons from different classes or who are using a second language. Similarly 'technical words' such as empathy, rapport, insight and defence mechanism are incomprehensible to many people. There are people in every locality who may use restrictive forms of language in their everyday communications.

Nurses deal with many people who use what Bernstein (1959) has called restricted code (public language in Chapter 3). Nurses, because of their occupational status, are encouraged to use elaborated code (formal language) because of the professional and medicotechnical influences on their role. In short, the client may not speak the same 'language' as the nurse and this can accentuate perceived class and cultural differences. Language is only one possible inhibition to the counselling process. Culture and gender differences between the nurse and the patient can cause differences in thinking, habits, values and beliefs. Occasionally these can be insurmountable and referral is the only course of action.

Many patients or clients are physically unwell. They may be fatigued, confused, malaised or unconscious. The over-enthusiastic nurse counsellor must remember that counselling can be too taxing for many who are really ill. This does not mean that counselling skills cannot find some general use in all nursing contexts. It is only a matter of being sensitive to all of the person's needs and recognizing when rigorous counselling is inappropriate.

The issue of trust has a two-way influence on the nurse and the counselling relationship. Trust achieved in counselling can be carried over to other situations in which the nurse and patient come together. The reverse is also true. Counselling helps the nurse and patient get to know each other better, when opportunities to do this in many hospital and community settings are lacking.

A final point relates to the nurse's uniform. This can be a barrier to communication because it constantly reminds the client of the formal and institutional position of the nurse. It may also be a symbolic reminder of certain stereotypes of nurses such as 'nurse knows best', 'nurses are always busy', 'he or she is only doing her job', 'nurses are only concerned with physical illness' or 'nurses must report everything'. The uniform can communicate many things about the nurse counsellor before she even opens her mouth. The distancing effect of uniform is not easy for the nurse to deal with because, in many practice settings, uniforms are necessary for safety, protection and identification. There are, however, occasions when the uniform can be discarded in favour of other clothing and the nurse should bear this in mind on those occasions when it is possible to do so.

SUPPORT FOR THE NURSE COUNSELLOR

It is essential to remember that the nurse cannot learn or carry out the sometimes arduous task of counselling without support from others. The nurse, no matter how expert, should have someone as mentor with whom he or she can discuss his or her own problems, mistakes and conflicts. It is best if this mentor has more experience of counselling but it is also possible to obtain additional support from a peer. In both cases, the mentor will also be bound by the rules of confidence to the nurse and his or her client. Whether the nurse can find a counselling mentor or not there is one principle that should be borne in mind: this is that, in order to be effective and to preserve his or her own mental health, the nurse counsellor should always be willing to realise his or her own limitations and to seek help and advice from colleagues. If one wants to give help then one should be able to receive help. It is somewhat hypocritical to expect others to avail themselves of our help when we are unable to accept help ourselves. It is the hallmark of a professional to be human and to be able to compensate for human fallabilities. It is not possible to avoid personal problems, mistakes or conflicts, it is only possible to try to hide them and struggle alone.

REFLECTIVE ACTIVITIES

1. Write out a descriptive definition of counselling in about 200 words. Refer to the section on the definition of counselling.
2. Ask a friend to describe a day in his/her life at work in detail. Say that you are only going to listen. Try to keep the person talking for as long as possible using non-verbal behaviour and limiting anything you say to a single word. If you can enlist the help of another friend ask that person to observe you both. At the end of the activity ask each person to report on their observations. Begin with the speaker's report first the listener second and the observer last. You can repeat this activity by changing roles as speaker, listener and observer. You may also be able to think of different topics to talk about.
3. Repeat Activity 2 but try to keep the person talking by using reflecting, paraphrasing and summarizing.
4. Ask one of your peers who is not a close friend and who is also interested in developing counselling skill to tell you as much about himself or herself as possible. Just listen and without taking notes remember what he or she has said. At the end of her description, which should last 5–10 min or longer, report back on everything that you can remember. Ask the speaker to correct anything that

you have said or remind you of anything you have forgotten. Discuss the differences in what was said and what you heard.

5. Ask a friend who you trust and who trusts you, to share with you a secret, a recent worry, stress, a close relationship or a mistake. Repay this trust by doing the same. Look at the section on immediacy and discuss this in relationship to your sharing.

SELF-EVALUATION TASKS

1. Define the term 'counselling' in your own words.
2. List and briefly describe the three stages of Egan's model.
3. List the skills of the counsellor and the skills of the client.
4. Define the terms: rapport; genuineness; empathy; resistance; defence mechanism; and immediacy.
5. Carry out a counselling session using a real-life problem of one of your friends. Videotape the session and observe your performance. This is also a useful exercise for observing the real self as well as counselling performance.

Check your answers with the text where possible.

CHAPTER 8

Skills for social influence

LEARNING OBJECTIVES

You should concentrate on being able to:

1. Define the terms: motivation; intrinsic motivation; extrinsic motivation; drive reduction; operant conditioning; goal-directed behaviour; frustration; problem-solving.
2. List and briefly describe six steps in the process of motivating others.
3. Define the term 'teaching' in terms of facilitating learning.
4. List at least nine situations encountered in nursing that require teaching skill from the nurse.
5. List three stages of a 'teaching process', including under each stage those actions that enable the stage to be achieved.
6. Be able to describe learning outcomes using several different frameworks.
7. List and briefly describe 18 methods of learning that may be used for patients and learner nurses.
8. List at least 20 aids to learning that may be used in patient teaching.
9. List at least 10 methods for gaining and keeping attention during teaching.
10. List and briefly describe 10 principles for giving feedback when teaching.
11. Describe methods for evaluating the effect of learning.
12. Describe the special considerations required when teaching patients.
13. Define the term 'diversional technique'.
14. List at least 10 situations in which diversion may be useful in nursing practice.
15. List and briefly describe seven methods of diversion.
16. List seven 'considerations' when providing occupation.

SOCIAL INFLUENCE

The skills described here are really a loose collection of miscellaneous skills that have a common link in that they tend to influence other people's actions in accordance with the nurse's wishes. The nurse is encouraging the patient or other person to do what he or she wants rather than leaving the person to his or her own devices. This is not to say that all other skills mentioned in this text do not have any element of social influence. It is rather that in these skills the nurse's guidance and direction are more apparent. In Chapter 9, skills that extend beyond influence to more explicit control of others are discussed.

MOTIVATING OTHERS

Motivation is a word that essentially means 'reasons for behaviour'. The fundamental assumption is that every piece of human behaviour is carried out for a particular reason. The study of human motivation is concerned with these reasons for human actions. When we ask questions such as 'Why did she do that?' or 'I wonder what causes people to behave in this strange fashion' and when we make guesses about why people (including ourselves) do things, we are enquiring about human motivating factors.

A study of motivation helps the nurse to carry out two basic skills. The first is to assess a person's needs and motives. This is a basic prerequisite for many of the social skills described in this book. The second skill is providing reasons for others to do particular things, to incite action. There are many occasions when the nurse must encourage, provide incentive or give reasons for behaviour expected from the patient. The nurse must be able to get others to do things, whether they are patients, colleagues or subordinates. In order to motivate others the nurse must identify an appropriate type of motivation and then set up the motivational condition that is likely to bring about the required behaviour. Motivating factors may be divided into two main types, intrinsic and extrinsic. Intrinsic motivation involves causes that are part of the action being carried out, while for extrinsic motivation the causes are not part of the action.

Intrinsic Motivation

Intrinsic motivation covers those causes that emanate from the stimulus properties of the task itself. Just carrying out the task is cause enough to carry on. Hunt (1960) suggests very simply that incongruity between the person's present thoughts and skills and new tasks or problems will encourage the person to minimize the incongruity.

Some people actually grow to enjoy this and seek out situations in which this sort of incongruity occurs. When using approaches such as trying to get a person interested in a subject or making the learning material interesting, we are trying to make the task itself intrinsically motivating. Harlow (1950) found that monkeys would spend time over and over again solving the same puzzle device. There are many examples of puzzles that keep people occupied for hours on end. Rubik's Cube is a puzzle that has high intrinsic motivating properties. Many games are intrinsically motivating, particularly those that are less dependent on competition with others or some sort of material reward. Activities such as playing music (alone), reading, gardening and many hobbies are maintained by intrinsic motivation when people say that they do it because of enjoyment or just for the fun of it.

Extrinsic Motivation

Two of the most influential extrinsic motivation theories are drive-reduction theory (Hull, 1943) and operant conditioning (Skinner, 1953). In both cases the motivating factor is not a part of the action taken but, on completion of the activity, something is gained or some desirable state achieved.

Drive Reduction

Hull (1943) suggested that all behaviour resulted from the satisfaction of basic needs; these consisted of primary biological needs such as air, food, water, physical safety, optimum temperature, removal of waste products (excretion), rest and sexual reproduction. If any of these factors are lacking, a state of increased arousal and activity occurs, which is directed towards the restoration of this lack or imbalance. As the lack increases, a state of drive is produced. As the deficiency becomes more severe, drive is increased, which causes more activity to be directed towards meeting the needs. This could possibly explain why the starving or the severely dyspnoeic human becomes so single-minded in his or her efforts to solve the problem. While drive-reduction explains the causation of many human actions, it is not generally accepted that it is the origin of all behaviour as Clark Hull would suggest (Hunt, 1960). However, the nurse deals with many situations when primary biological needs must be met, and so this sort of motivating factor is of profound significance to the nurse.

Operant Conditioning

Skinner (1953) considers that the most important motivating factors are those concerned with the consequences of behaviour. Skinner concerns himself with observable behaviour only and says:

> Every science has at some time or other looked for causes of action inside the things it has studied. Sometimes the practice has proved useful, sometimes it has not. There is nothing wrong with an inner explanation as such, but events that are located inside a system are likely to be difficult to observe.
>
> *Skinner, 1953*

His persistent concern with observable behaviour has allowed us to consider an important range of motivating factors. Two features of operant conditioning are important, the 'operant' and the 'reinforcer'. The operant is an action or set of actions carried out by the organism, that are controlled consciously by it. Examples of human actions that may take the form of operants include speaking a word or a single body movement such as lifting a hand or winking an eye. A reinforcer is something that will increase the probability of the particular operant being repeated. Positive reinforcers are pleasurable and increase operant repetition when present. A common word for this is reward. Reinforcers have motivating properties, examples being food, money and social approval. Negative reinforcers cause operant repetition by their removal. Painful or distressing stimuli are often negative reinforcers. Take the example of a fairly common piece of behaviour (an operant) familiar to the nurse, such as asking for an analgesic. The patient asks for something to relieve the pain. The pain is an unpleasant persistent stimulus. The nurse provides the prescribed drug and the pain is removed. The patient associates the asking behaviour with a happy consequence and is more likely to ask again when the pain returns. The removal of pain has been negatively reinforcing. A concept similar to negative reinforcement is punishment. This involves the presentation of a stimulus after the action that decreases the likelihood of its being repeated.

Many consequences of human behaviour such as pain, deprivation or social disapproval obviously control behaviour. Some forms of punishment and negative reinforcement are morally unacceptable for nursing. It is the anticipation of the consequence of the behavioural action that is motivating to the human being. Most forms of gambling such as fruit machines, betting, bingo and roulette are effective in maintaining participation of the gambler because of reinforcement, which is fairly consistent but unpredictable. These rewards and punishments constitute a third category of causes of behaviour. The main possible categories of human motivation are summarized in Figure 8.1.

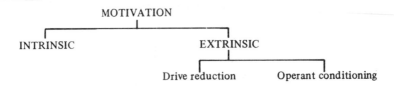

Figure 8.1 Theories of motivation.

A final point about motives should be borne in mind. If a type of motivation is to be selected by the nurse, it must be something valued or seen as important by the other person. If it is not relevant it will be worthless.

Goal-directed Behaviour

When we wish to motivate others, we are often setting goals for the other person. The goal involves gaining something or achieving some favoured state of affairs (Weiner, 1989; Baron, 1992). The goal is usually set in the future and may be described in behavioural terms. One of the important features of the nursing process is goal-setting. When a goal is stated, one usually adopts a model that sees the person moving from an unacceptable state of affairs on a journey of change towards the goal. Interruption of this journey can result in several phenomena commonly referred to in this text. **Frustration** is a term used to describe the emotion experienced by the person when the 'route' to the goal is blocked. Sometimes a less-direct route can be taken, but the person will be frustrated until the obstacle to goal achievement has been surmounted. Removal of the barrier will, in itself, have motivating properties. A blocking of the direct route to a goal has also been described as a **problem**. Working out an alternative way of achieving the goal is then known as problem-solving.

Imagine that two solutions to the problem are available, both equally attractive but which cannot be carried out together. If the person cannot progress because he does not know which one to choose, this could be described as **conflict**. Conflict is also a state that causes frustration.

Some goals are, by their nature, difficult or impossible for the person to achieve. Two important principles arise from this. First, the goals that are set should be realistic and attainable. The second principle involves the idea of intermediate goals. Sometimes the difficult goal can be met by setting a series of sub-goals, which, when achieved, make the final step towards achieving the goal much easier.

Often goals must be set by the nurse, although sometimes they may be set by the patient or by both parties. The latter is clearly most acceptable. A goal set by the nurse becomes an expectation imposed by another person on the patient. Patients often but not always accept these.

Practical Motivating

The final activity for motivating others involves setting up the conditions or stimuli to provide the particular motivating factors. Many skills described in this text will be used. The most important are set induction, explanation, giving feedback, gaining rapport, respect, genuineness, force-field analysis and offering alternative frames of reference.

In conclusion the points given in this discussion will be summarized to give a simplified version of a process for motivating others:

1. Identify the desired behaviour.
2. Set realistic and appropriate goals.
3. Set intermediate goals if necessary.
4. Identify appropriate motivating factors.
5. Select and use social skills that will set up the motivating conditions.
6. Evaluate the effects of motivational action and adapt.

TEACHING

Teaching will be taken here to mean an activity that helps others to learn. A fairly restrictive definition of teaching emphasizes the passing on of skills, knowledge or opinions by one person to another. This approach to teaching imposes certain limitations on the learner if strictly adhered to. The first is that passing on and giving tend to insinuate some degree of passivity in the learner. It is a common phenomenon in many areas of education to find learners who say that they could not learn because they have not covered the topic in a teaching session, i.e. they have not been 'given' the knowledge. This suggests that the learner has no control over information or skill discovery. A second problem with this definition is that the one person giving to another necessitates the supposition that the teacher is a subject-matter expert, an only source of the material to be learned. The teacher must then not make mistakes and must never be wrong. Few teachers are experts in all areas of their subject and few are infallible. The third point about the giving approach to learning is that logically the learner can only extract the skills and knowledge that the teacher possesses at any one time. The learner is then limited by the knowledge, skills, memory, attitudes, moods and inclinations of the teacher or group of teachers. Learners should be allowed to surpass the ability of teachers if they are capable, both on specific topics and skills and in the area of special skill and knowledge as a whole.

As a result, teaching is best seen as the activity of engineering environments in which others can learn. Whether one provides information, helps to identify problems or provides motivation, feedback, relevance, simplicity and understanding, teaching is facilitating learning rather than doing everything for the learner. This latter point may be naively obvious but it is traditionally forgotten or ignored. Indeed, it is a modern trend to see the teacher as a facilitator of learning and often the term 'facilitator' is preferred to that of teacher in a move to develop student-centredness in learning (ENB, 1987; Burnard, 1992).

Learning is best defined as 'change in behaviour or behavioural potential brought about by experience'. The fact that we perceive the world throughout our waking life suggests that learning takes place at all times. Two important points about teaching and intentional learning qualify the common preconception of learning as an activity separated from other life experiences. The common belief about learning is that it improves knowledge and skills for the better. Learning, however, can be for the worse. Training courses and teaching tend to concern themselves with changes advantageous to the learner. The second common orientation to teaching is that it is concerned with particular changes and others are not considered. Teaching and learning are generally concerned with directed intentional changes in specific areas. This is the basic foodstuff of the curriculum, course plan and learning objectives. All other learning (i.e. life) generally has no importance to the teacher and learner. Teaching and learning as we understand the words are generally concerned with specified experiences and behaviour changes.

A word about behaviour change would perhaps be useful at this stage. Behaviour includes body movements and spoken words alike. The ability to think out a problem and voice a possible solution is behavioural, just as much as walking or riding a bicycle. Take one example: a learner is asked the question, 'What is the eighth cranial nerve?' and he or she cannot answer. The teacher says 'the auditory nerve'. Here a learning experience, the sound of the correct response, has been given. One would expect that the learner stores this response in memory. On subsequent occasions, he or she will repeat the response when the question is asked again. Here behavioural ability has changed, just as much as in the case of the nurse who can give an intramuscular injection, when prior to the course of learning he or she could not.

When nurses are teaching they are bringing about a change in the other person that they believe necessary or valuable. The nurse may be a teacher in several situations and it is useful to describe some of the most common:

1. Patients who need to learn the nature of illness and know how to cope with it.
2. Patients who need to learn self-application of therapy. Dietary control, subcutaneous injection and control of anxiety and urine testing provide some examples of this.
3. Patients who need to relearn activities of daily living. Sometimes the patient needs to learn once again to dress, wash, cook, walk and even communicate with others.
4. Patients who need to learn social skills. They may need to learn how to establish and keep human contact and co-operate with others in an acceptable way.
5. Patients who need to learn to co-operate in treatments and procedures.
6. Student and pupil nurses to meet needs for state examinations and qualifications.
7. Job instruction for all employees. As a manager, the nurse will need to teach others how to do the work required of them. This is necessary for efficiency and safety at work.
8. Health education. In hospital and the community, people are taught to prevent illness and disorder, e.g. through breast examination, diet, avoidance of hazards.
9. Relatives who need to learn and administer nursing or first aid to family members with persistent disorders, e.g. epilepsy.

Outline of Teaching Skill

The skill of teaching will be taken as a three-stage process involving the activities summarized below:

1. Planning:
   (a) Deciding the purpose.
   (b) Assessing the learner.
   (c) Identifying the content.
   (d) Writing objectives.
   (e) Selecting learning methods.
   (f) Selecting aids or assistance.
2. Action:
   (a) Gaining attention.
   (b) Motivating to learn.
   (c) Giving feedback.
   (d) Encouraging practice, rehearsal, revision.
   (e) Presenting information.

3. Evaluating:
   (a) Pencil-and-paper testing.
   (b) Assessing skills.
   (c) Self-reporting.
   (d) Questioning.

This list is given as an overview so that each of the actions can be discussed in detail. It is possible to suggest three areas for a teaching nursing care plan: (i) purpose; (ii) resources; and (iii) learner objectives (Zander *et al.*, 1978; Rotam and Abbatt, 1982). The work by Zander *et al.* will also prove useful to the reader because it provides a whole range of examples of plans for teaching patients.

Planning

Deciding the Purpose

A statement of purpose encourages the nurse to think about why the teaching and learning is required. The nurse makes a decision about what the patient or learner needs – what is required or beneficial. Sometimes teaching sessions are carried out for reasons other than helping others to learn. In the case of the nurse the reason may be to be examined (e.g. with ward-based assessments), to practise teaching, because he or she likes the subject or wants to try a new teaching method.

When deciding the purpose of the learning experience it is useful to know what people can learn. The most common areas of learning are described as knowledge, attitudes and psychomotor skills. Knowledge (or cognitive) learning involves memorizing and recalling information, facts and relationships between information and fact. It involves bringing to mind the required material. Attitude-learning involves feelings and predispositions towards ideas. It includes likes and dislikes, acceptance of ideas and willingness to perceive information. Psychomotor-skill learning is concerned with the area of carrying out particular actions. Examples of this type of learning are extremely practical, such as riding a bicycle, setting a trolley or giving an injection. More detail on these areas of learning will be given under the heading of objective writing. In brief, the nurse should ask, 'Do I want the learner to know something, change his or her attitudes or to be able to something?'.

Describing Learning Outcomes

One of the important skills in teaching is to be able to describe learning outcomes and help the learner to describe learning outcomes. This is necessary so that the teacher practitioner can draw up a learning programme, agree a learning contract with the learner and make explicit the learning that has occurred. It must be remembered that sometimes the learner may be able to describe learning retroactively as well as proactively.

There are two approaches to describing learning outcomes, the behavioural objectives approach and the experiential approach (ENB, 1987). The learning objectives approach to learning identifies the learning outcome before entering into the learning experience. In this approach, a learning session without objectives is similar to a mystery tour or a day's outing to a place known only to the organizer. Imagine that only one person knows where the holiday destination will be. Several problems will be apparent. First the would-be daytripper may arrive at a place that he or she neither likes nor wants to be. Secondly, the daytripper does not know where he or she is supposed to be until the very last minute, only picking up vague clues when travelling along. A third problem is that, should the organizer become fatally ill, nobody would know where they were supposed to go. Finally, because the organizer is the only person who knows the goal, all the occupants of the coach, the daytrippers and the driver are dependent on the organizer. Their actions are governed by him or her (i.e. leaving the bus, what to take on the journey, the route the driver takes).

Learning without objectives is comparable with this mystery tour. The learner does not know what he or she is doing, why he or she is doing it or when he or she has achieved the goal. In fact, the goals have not been set up.

Instructional objectives achieve the following functions:

1. They tell the learner what he or she is expected to learn and eliminate uncertainty and confusion.
2. They guide the actions of the teacher.
3. They dictate teaching method.
4. They dictate the evaluation process.
5. They encourage both teacher and learner to make decisions and to clarify the whole learning experience.

The achievement of these functions depends on the quality of the written objective. According to Mager (1962) an objective is a statement of intent. Three components of an instructional objective should be present. When formulating an objective the nurse should:

1. Identify the terminal behaviour by name and specify the kind of behaviour that will be accepted as evidence that the learner has achieved the objective.
2. Define the desired behaviour by describing the important conditions under which the behaviour will be expected to occur.

3. Specify the criteria of acceptable performance by describing how well the learner must perform to be considered acceptable.

An objective describes the outcome and behaviour. It is not merely a description or summary of content, since it states what the learner should be able to do and how acceptability will be measured. A crucial point is that the objective should describe observable behaviour, not covert phenomena such as knowing, appreciating or being aware. Two objectives, one theoretical and one practical, may serve to demonstrate the instructional objective:

1. 'The learner will be able to list and explain 13 key concepts of leadership as described by Grohar-Murray and DiGroce (1992) in a pencil and paper test within 30 min.'
2. 'The learner will be able to explain to a patient on a ward the actions required by him or her while passing a nasogastric tube, so that no problem occurs that is associated with the patient not knowing what to do.'

A learning session may consist of one or several objectives. Four is usually the average optimum number of objectives that can be achieved in a 45-min teaching/learning session. Each objective is specific to a particular point, item of knowledge or unit of skill or change. To be able to write objectives one needs to be aware of the content of the learning experience. In addition, the item of learning is defined by the level of learning required. These are described in the form of educational or learning domains. The lists that follow are given as examples to assist an understanding of the range of learning levels. The first three domains are the most popular in educational circles; they are not, however, the only way of categorizing objectives in terms of the ability achieved. They are described in terms of knowledge, attitude or skill learning.

A taxonomy of educational objectives is as follows (source: cognitive domain adapted from Bloom (1956); affective domain adapted from Karthwohl *et al.* (1964); psychomotor domain adapted from Simpson (1966)):

1. **Cognitive domain:**
   1.0 Knowledge: recalling, remembering, retrieving facts, ideas, details.
   2.0 Comprehension: understanding, translation, interpretation, extrapolation.
   3.0 Application: the ability to use facts, principles and theories.
   4.0 Analysis: the ability to break down facts, information and ideas.
   5.0 Synthesis: the ability to build elements of a body of knowledge into an understandable whole.

6.0 Evaluation: assess the value, merit, reliability of information, principles and methods.

2. **Affective domain:**

1.0 Receiving: willingness to receive an idea or suggestion.

2.0 Responding: accepting an idea by acting upon it.

3.0 Valuing: accepting the worth of an idea, accepting it in preference to others.

4.0 Organization: conceptualizing a value, relating it to other values.

5.0 Characterization by a value complex: accepting the value to such an extent that it is predictable and characteristic of that person.

3. **Psychomotor domain:**

1.0 Perception: awareness of the sensory input of salient features of the skill.

2.0 Set: physical and psychological readiness to initiate the required action.

3.0 Guided response: intentional actions carried out with caution and conscious control.

4.0 Mechanism: action established in behavioural repertoire and carried out confidently.

5.0 Complex overt response: performing with ease, action becomes automatic because of well-established pathways between perceptual and motor activity.

Another taxonomy listed below, that is not so established as that presented in the list above, serves to demonstrate a different approach to categorizing learning objectives. It is a taxonomy of experiential objectives and is particularly relevant to patient and nursing learning.

The categories of the experiential taxonomy by Steinaker and Bell (1975) are as follows:

1.0 **Exposure**. Consciousness of an experience. This involves two kinds of exposure and a readiness for further experience:

1.1 Sensory.

1.2 Response.

1.3 Readiness.

2.0 **Participation**. The decision to become physically a part of an experience. There are two levels of interaction within this category concerned with reproduction and alteration of the material:

2.1 Representation.

2.2 Modification.

3.0 **Identification**. As the participant modifies the experience, the process of identification with the experience begins. There are four levels of experience within this category:

3.1 Reinforcement.
3.2 Emotional.
3.3 Personal.
3.4 Sharing.
4.0 **Internalization**. The participant moves from identification to internalization when the experience begins to affect the lifestyle of the participant. There are two levels within this category:
4.1 Expansion.
4.2 Intrinsic.
5.0 **Dissemination**. The experience moves beyond internalization to the dissemination of the experience. It goes beyond positive sharing which began at level 3.0 and involves two levels:
5.1 Informational.
5.2 Homiletic.

Transferable Personal Skills

A second approach to describing learning is the transferable skills approach. In essence, this is particularly useful where the nurses see that they may be facilitating learning that is useful in other aspects of life in addition to the current learning situation. The following describes a list of learning outcomes that are particularly relevant to the preparatory and continuing education of nurses (adapted from Hind, 1989):

- learning and study skills;
- vocal communication skills;
- non-verbal communication skills;
- written communication skills;
- data-handling and presentation skills;
- interview skills;
- presentation skills;
- selling and negotiating skills;
- personal skills;
- group work skills;
- thinking skills;
- information-gathering skills;
- consultancy skills.

From Novice to Expert

Another approach to describing learning outcomes is related to levels of learning related to professional practice. Benner (1984) describes the following levels of learning for the nurse practitioner.

1. Graded qualitative distinctions – comparing various personal judgements that are made in patient care situations in the same issue.

2. Common meanings – developing shared understanding about common nursing care situations.
3. Assumptions, expectations and sets – these are commonalities that enable the nurse to predict what will happen next in a given situation or context.
4. Paradigm cases and personal knowledge – the use of past concrete situations as examples on which to determine practice in a similar future situation.
5. Maxims – these are the assumed self-evident truths or facts about a situation that are self-evident to the experienced or expert practitioner but not to others.
6. Unplanned practices – some aspects of the nurse's work are not part of the usual role of the nurse but nurses adopt them out of necessity or interest. In turn, these practices are handed on from nurse to nurse and become an established part of nursing work in a specific practice environment.

Selecting Learning Methods

Once the objectives have been identified, it is possible to select the appropriate experience to help the learner to achieve the objective. These experiences are commonly called teaching or learning methods. The methods available for patient and nurse teaching are listed below with a brief description of each.

1. Explanation. Spoken description or information given, usually on a one-to-one basis in everyday personal interaction.
2. Lecture. Usually teacher-centred and teacher-directed presentation of a fairly substantial amount of information to a medium-to-large group of people usually taking at least 30 min or longer.
3. Lecturette. A relatively new term describing a lecture to a small group or one person taking 5–30 min covering one or two objectives.
4. Free group discussion. Discussion on a particular topic in a group of 3–12 people. Amount of participation and route to learning unpredictable. Teacher participates as an equal. Course of discussion determined by group members.
5. Directed group discussion. A free discussion where the teacher directs the flow of conversation and topics and issues raised.
6. Demonstration. Performing a skill for another to observe. Usually performed by teacher at normal speed then repeated, broken down into constituent parts and at a slower speed. Usually appropriate to technical skills.
7. Modelling. By their very actions the teachers' attitudes, beliefs and social behaviours are passed on because of the learner's inclination

to imitate or identify with those people respected, admired or seen as expert. This method is usually appropriate to social skills and attitudes. It is a very common method of learning in nursing but often forgotten.

8. Running commentary. It is common in some craft occupations and advanced skills learning (e.g. driving) for skilled practitioners to demonstrate the skill to a learner by speaking out loud the observations thoughts and decisions they are making while carrying out the skill. This is particularly useful in enabling the learner to understand the decision-making processes that accompany skilled action. It can also be adopted by the student to facilitate reflective thinking and as a means of evaluating skill performance. It is not easy to do and requires some practice.

9. Briefing and de-briefing. This method involves the discussion of a learning experience, its objectives, processes and constraints before it is undertaken, and the evaluation of learning afterwards. It is suggested that briefing and de-briefing should take as much time, if not more than the actual experience itself. The method promotes reflective thinking and student empowerment (White and Ewan; 1991; Pearson and Smith, 1985). Counselling skills are particularly useful for this activity.

10. Simulated experience. This involves learning using representations of reality and takes the form of gaming, role-acting, simulation machines and models. It re-enacts the essential properties of real life in a safe environment where dangerous consequences are removed. It also allows time and the scale of a situation to be manipulated (e.g. in ward management or when injecting an orange).

11. Reflective journals. This is a method that uses principles similar to keeping a diary and encourages reflective thinking and provides a personal record of learning and achievement (Powell, 1985).

12. Project work. A planned method of inquiry organized to solve a problem or elicit information or discovery learning. This is similar to the research method (Adderly et al., 1975).

13. Seminar. This is a class that meets for systematic study under the direction of a leader or organizer. It differs from a lecture in that participation from all members is expected and information comes from all, not just the teacher.

14. Reading. This is frequently acknowledged but often forgotten. It requires basic abilities in the learner to understand language, interpret written form and possess a broad enough vocabulary. The willingness of learner to read is obviously crucial.

15. Workshop. This is similar to a seminar but members tend to participate in a craft or activity while sharing ideas and skills with peers.

16. Observation. This involves watching others in the course of their activities from the sideline.
17. Participant observation. This is watching others in their activities while being involved as an active participant.
18. Counselling. The counselling process encourages the client to learn the nature of his or her problems and how to overcome them.

Identification of learning resources

The identification of learning resource is an important role of the practitioner teacher (ENB, 1987; Gillies, 1989). Resources for learning take the form of a variety of stimulus materials, which help the learner to acquire the required knowledge or skill, motivate the learner or increase the modes of reception. Examples of visual resources are:

- motion films;
- video television;
- photographic slides;
- photographs (prints);
- overhead projections;
- epidiascope projections;
- diagrams;
- charts;
- handouts (language in print);
- books;
- magazines;
- pamphlets;
- models;
- equipment and machines;
- the surrounding environment – people and objects;
- microscope;
- blackboards, whiteboards;
- computer displays;
- self.

Examples of auditory resources are:

- sound-tape playback;
- records;
- stethoscopes;
- the surrounding environment;
- electronically-synthesized sound;
- radio;
- telephone;
- sound feedback of the galvanic skin response;
- the human voice.

Examples of tactile resources are:

- equipment-handling ;
- the texture of objects;
- other human beings (palpation);
- self.

Examples of olfactory resources include:

- human excretions and discharges, e.g. urine;
- chemicals, e.g. acetone;
- the surrounding environment;
- food.

Finally, gustatory resources comprise foodstuffs.

Resources should always be meticulously produced and must have a purpose (i.e. they should be chosen to meet a need). They should be clear and vivid enough to stimulate the sense organs and cause effective perception. Whenever possible, aids should be simple rather than complicated.

Selection of assistants involves deciding on help that may be required of others – colleagues, patients or people from other disciplines. It may be useful to use two teachers when there are too many things to do. There could be a need for participation when tasks cannot be carried out alone, e.g. lifting and carrying patients.

Teaching Skills in Action

Understanding the learner's needs

This involves making decisions about the learner's ability to learn and what he or she already knows. Ability assessment will consist of a rough estimation of the person's intellectual ability and personal characteristics. The other major area of assessment is the learner's previous relevant knowledge and skills. Assessing the learner is crucial at this point because it influences both the selection of content and the nature of the learning objectives.

Often an understanding of the learner's needs and the possibility of meeting these needs is achieved by the negotiation of a learning contract between teacher and learner. In essence, the learning contract is an agreement between both parties about what should be achieved and how it is best achieved (Mazhindu, 1990).

The issue of facilitating the learners' personal involvement and responsibility for their own learning has been promoted in recent years by developing student self-direction. Several ways of developing this in nursing practice have been suggested (Mast and Van Atta, 1986):

1. Build in opportunities for learners to be self-directed and responsible and to exercise their own individual learning styles and preferences.
2. Encourage learners to use their current experiences as a resource for their own and others' learning.
3. Select learning material that will be applied to life tasks.
4. Create a problem-centred rather than a subject-centred orientation to learning.

Several other skills are relevant to teaching skill in the practice setting. They include: (i) gaining and keeping attention; (ii) motivating the learner; (iii) giving feedback; (iv) encouraging rehearsal and revision; and (v) presentation skills.

Gaining and Keeping Attention

Set-induction skills will prove useful for gaining and keeping the learner's attention. The following methods are useful for teaching skills (adapted from Hargie *et al.*, 1987):

1. The use of novel stimuli. Audiovisual aids can be used to achieve this method of set induction.
2. Posing an intriguing problem.
3. Making a controversial or provocative statement.
4. Unusual or unexpected teacher behaviour.
5. Provision of comforts. A comfortable environment and satisfying any needs for food, drink or relief from discomfort can help to keep learner's attention.
6. Personal attributes of the participants. The learner's impression of the teacher's skill, efficiency and personality attributes may all affect the learner's willingness to receive information or assistance from a teacher.
7. Prior instructions. Just telling the learner what he or she is expected to do helps to gain and keep attention. One important way of giving instructions is to present a simple outline of the learning experience or procedure.
8. Reviewing previous information. In addition to gaining attention, this refreshes the learner's memory and assists in demonstrating the relevance of the new information.
9. Outlining the functions. Objectives give information on the functions of the session.
10. Outlining the goals. Again objectives can perform this function but broader aims and purposes may be introduced to achieve this effect.
11. Educational set. Siegel and Siegel (1965) suggest that learners may be prepared to receive 'factual' or 'conceptual' information at the

outset (or beginning) of the learning session. The resulting 'factual set' or 'conceptual set' of the learner will influence his or her attitude to the learning experience. This will have its greatest effect if the teacher's presentation and the learner's educational set match.

Motivating the Learner

To encourage and maintain active learning one can take two broad approaches. One is to discover the needs of the learner and meet them. The second is to make the teaching session motivating in itself. The former uses the principle of extrinsic motivation, the latter intrinsic motivation. All human beings are influenced by several different motives at different times and at any one time. Motivational influences change from one moment to the next. The aim of the teacher is to maximize those motives that are conducive to achieving the learning objectives and minimize those that interfere with the learning process. One important aspect of 'motivating to learn' is reinforcement by rewarding appropriate learner behaviour and ignoring or punishing behaviour inconsistent with the required learning. Punishment does not mean violence or severe psychological harm. Any behaviour such as disapproval, poor test marks and disagreement expressed by a teacher can be considered punitive.

Giving Feedback

Learning is a concept that has embodied change in some form or other. Furthermore, the person is undergoing desirable change in a specific area determined by each instructional objective. Learning can be viewed as an adjustment to a more desirable state. Feedback is a concept borrowed from information theory that describes a situation in which an object undergoing change receives information about the change process, thus helping that object to judge the effectiveness of its change. A thermostat is the classical example of a machine that provides self-regulation. This idea of feedback has been applied to human beings and it describes those situations in which the person receives information about himself or herself and the changes that he or she is undergoing.

The skill of providing feedback is fundamental to all social skills. It is inevitable that it will occur when two human beings engage in communicative transactions between each other. When feedback is given, it does not automatically mean that the person will act on it and this is a fundamental difference between human systems and mechanical systems, i.e. that the former are not automatic. Lewis (1973) has also described another phenomenon that makes human feedback systems unusual. The phenomenon is called 'action-reaction interdependence'. In simple terms, one person performs an action, the other reacts to it and thus gives feedback. The first person then adjusts his or her subsequent behaviour and this influences the type of feedback he or she will receive. Feedback in interpersonal relationships is cyclic and dynamic. It helps us to be aware of what we do and how we do it and several principles may be followed to improve the quality of intentional feedback:

1. Feedback should be given in the form of description rather than an evaluation. Opinions, value judgements and guesses about the learner's motives are rarely helpful.
2. It should be constructive, not destructive. It should help the learner, not limit or restrict him.
3. It should be specific. Vague terminology or indirect reference to the behaviour in question tends to leave the learner in limbo. Feedback should be relevant and direct.
4. Feedback should be given about those aspects that are capable of change. If the person can really do nothing about the behaviour or attribute in question it will only cause conflict and emotional tension.
5. Feedback should be tactful and given in a climate of genuine concern and caring for the other person.
6. Reference to the behaviour should be made rather than reference to the person.
7. Feedback should be given at the person's request, not imposed upon him or her.
8. It should not normally always be one-sided. The teacher should allow the learner the opportunity to give feedback about the teacher's behaviour.
9. Feedback should be immediate and not delayed. It has reinforcing and motivating properties.
10. Feedback should be accurate and consistent. Over the long term, inconsistent feedback from one person can be unsettling for the learner.

Encourage Rehearsal and Revision

A simple point, which has profound effects on learning, involves two principles: (i) allow active participation; and (ii) encourage stimulating repetition. Learning is seated in experience and this means that the learner must use the knowledge or skills to retain them.

Even something simple, like allowing the learner to 'have a go' after a procedure has been demonstrated, is often forgotten. Revision of knowledge merely means consciously recalling and manipulating the thoughts and facts. In this way, they are more effectively retained. The issue of active rather than passive learning is important only because passive participation by learners in many fields of education is common and permitted. The nurse who teaches patients should never forget that the nature of the nursing relationship makes patient participation unavoidable, let alone necessary, if effective patient learning is to occur. Repetition should never be allowed to cause boredom or it will interfere with learning. Remember the saying attributed to Confucius: 'one seeing is worth one thousand hearings, one doing is worth one thousand seeings'.

Presentation of Information

Many teaching and learning situations are concerned with the presentation of information. Much of the earlier discussion on explanation is applicable here. Information presentation should be clear, ordered, concise and relevant. Wherever possible, information should be presented in more than one way and should be left with the learner in some permanent form (e.g. notes, handouts or references to literature). Presentation of information by the teacher will depend on speech skill, writing skill, ability to achieve rapport and organizational ability.

Demonstration is a form of information presentation that differs from the lecture and explanation. It is often concerned with psychomotor skill, and actions are an important component. Demonstration is common in patient teaching and the following sequence is suggested to provide a guide to the nurse who teaches by demonstration:

1. Give a short introductory talk, gain rapport, state objectives, provide links with previous material and other learning.
2. Demonstrate whole procedures at normal speed by a skilled person. No commentary is necessary.
3. Ask the learner(s) to describe the important points and what was observed. Encourage questions.
4. Demonstrate again, slowly and in smaller appropriate parts. The teaching plan will consist of a skill analysis where the skill is broken down into smaller units to facilitate comprehension, observation and skill acquisition. Explanation can be given at this stage and may take the form of a running commentary. Encourage questions.
5. Allow the learner(s) to have an attempt under supervision. Allow questions.
6. The learner should then demonstrate the skill to others at least once to gain feedback (from teacher or other students). Allow questions.
7. Plan for as much practice as possible, under supervision at first until competent. In the case of learner nurses, supervision is expected at all times.

This idea is also given support by the information processing model of training that suggests that all learning sessions can be organized around an input, action and feedback model (Stammers and Patrick, 1975). This essentially encourages us to think of three aspects of skill acquisition:

1. Recognizing when the skill activities should be brought into play.
2. Being proficient at the activities and the sequencing of activities required for adequate performance.
3. Evaluating the effect/consequences of activities and making the decision when to stop the skilled action sequence.

Evaluating Learning

It is traditionally the teacher's responsibility to assess how effective learning has been. The learner can, however, use most evaluative techniques to gain feedback without the help of others. Evaluation helps both the teacher and the learner to operate more effectively. The most common form of evaluation is the pencil-and-paper test. The teacher usually formulates questions that the learner must respond to. The ingenious learner can devise his or her own questions by setting them before the learning experience. Questions can also be set for oneself as information is collected or read. The important principle for testing in the latter situation is to allow a long period of time between question-setting and answering. When setting oneself questions it is best to be objective, very strict and honest. The topics covered should be those found most difficult and should be taken equally from all parts of the range of material. A variation on the self-administered pencil-and-paper test is the self-report on learning progress. This is often subjective and only approaches objectivity when the teacher uses efficient questioning, counselling or interviewing skills. Questioning skill, both spoken and written, is crucial to efficient teacher evaluation of learning and the teaching nurse should understand the pitfalls of questioning before engaging in this form of testing. One form of evaluation particularly suitable for skill learning is demonstration. The learner performs the skill and the teacher observes checking the performance with a criterion sheet. The criterion sheet describes the important parts of the skill and the measure of adequate performance. It is clear that instructional objectives are a crucial feature of learning evaluation. They provide assessment criteria and when used they make the job of evaluation more objective and much easier. Once again the importance of counselling in the process of evaluating learning cannot be underestimated. It is useful because it is a means of self-reporting undertaken in the context of a non-threatening relationship.

Evaluation is of little importance unless subsequent action is taken. Both the teacher and the learner should take corrective action on the basis of evaluative feedback. Both parties should actively participate. It is not satisfactory for the teacher to place all the responsibility for action on the learner or *vice versa*.

Teaching Patients

All of the previous discussion has relevance to the teaching of patients as much as to the teaching of other nurses. Nurses help patients to learn in a variety of ways. How to cope with illness, how to behave in hospital, how to cope on discharge and how to carry out procedures are just a selection of the areas in which nurses help patients learn. Teaching is an instrument of potential control, power and additional dependence because of the dependent relationship of the patient to the nurse. The nurse's expertise in teaching in this way takes on added importance.

Several factors in patient teaching should be borne in mind. The first difference between patient learning and student learning is that patients are suffering some form of illness or dysfunction and, as such, their ability to concentrate and participate is influenced by the degree of ill health. Some patients are completely unaware and unresponsive to their surroundings (e.g. the unconscious patient). With some patients it is difficult to assess the amount of awareness (e.g. the stuperosed, the demented, the confused and some mentally ill or handicapped people). Others are unresponsive and it is not possible to know if they are aware. Those coming out of unconsciousness, those in a catatonic state or those who are withdrawn or preoccupied do not give the impression that they can learn. Attempts to help patients learn should not be given up in these situations, rather nurses should alter their approach and not depend on the quality of patient feedback. Other patients may be fatigued or malaised and this will alter their ability to concentrate and comprehend. Nurse will need to judge the state of the patients and not overtax them. Short effective spans are better than long ineffective teaching sessions. Time can be wasted by ignoring these basic points.

Patients also come from a wide range of classes, abilities and experiences. Nurses will need to be adaptable as teachers to ensure that they reach each of their patients. It is no good treating those with poor intellect as if they are knowledgeable or treating those of high intellectual ability as if they are stupid. The responsibility for flexibility is with the nurse, not with the patient.

One final point should be made before leaving this discussion on helping others to learn. It is a common phenomenon, and apparently a natural inclination of some nurses, to take particular pride in their need to give knowledge or skills. This very often betrays itself in the adoption of a 'teacher' role. An example of this is when the ward sister stops everything to 'do some teaching'. When we begin to act 'the teacher' we have to accept everything that tends to go with it. Some people have had poor experiences of learning and will react with a negative attitude if the nurse appears to adopt the teacher image while relinquishing his or her other roles. Others will expect the teacher to be perfect and blame the teacher for mistakes. Yet others will wonder 'What gives you the right to be the teacher with me?'. These responses are likely to occur when one adopts a stereotyped teacher approach. Helping people to learn, particularly in the field of nursing, is not related to the mortar board, blackboard and tester image. Teaching can be extremely subtle, insidious and appropriate to ongoing nursing activities. The teaching nurse should be aware, skilled and adaptable. In this way, he or she will be able to take opportunities to teach as they arise rather than having to create them artificially.

DIVERSIONAL TECHNIQUE

Diversion in this context is the activity of directing a person's attention away from particular stimuli, preoccupying thoughts or unpleasant sensations and feelings. It is conducted on the assumption that these concerns are harmful or detrimental to the patient's progress.

Knowledge fundamental to practising the skill of diversion includes an understanding of perception, attention and motivation theory. This knowledge will assist the nurse in identifying situations in which diversion will be necessary. Diversional technique may be necessary in several conditions experienced by patients. These include:

- pain;
- thought disorder;
- delusion;
- obsessional thought;
- compulsive thought and action;
- depression;
- hallucination;
- bereavement;
- disordered self-image;
- grief;
- fear and anxiety;
- unusual body sensations;
- crisis;
- aggression and violence.

In all of these situations, the nurse will need to be sure that diversion will be the best course of action. Sometimes it is necessary to take advantage of problems such as bereavement and anxiety to help the patient develop in some way. Take, for instance, anxiety, which can be motivating. At times, the patient may need counselling or teaching to help him or her to learn how to cope with those things that cause concern. Diverting attention is just one method of preventing the patient's preoccupation causing him or her further harm. Diversion is really a stop-gap measure helping the patient to avoid harm. Long-term therapy will be necessary to remedy the cause to any lasting degree.

Before commencing diversional techniques, it will be necessary to identify the harmful feature and make sure that the cause cannot be removed. The nurse can use several skills described in this text and, in particular, methods to achieve set induction will help to divert a patient's attention.

Presenting a novel sensory stimulus

Strong sensory stimuli or unusual stimuli may capture the person's attention. Providing books or television programmes that interest the patient may help to divert attention. Bright objects or toys may divert a child's attention. The presentation of novel stimuli may at least prevent boredom. Boredom will allow preoccupation with body sensations and thoughts. A change of environment can have the same effect.

Posing an intriguing problem

This is a set-induction method, which can create diversion by absorbing the patient in the problem.

Making a controversial or provocative statement

This tends to be emotionally motivating. Carefully used, this may encourage the patient to become absorbed in social transaction.

Conversation

This tends to provide distraction because the patient, once involved, will be occupied in giving attention and verbal reply, both activities requiring some degree of concentration. The nurse should ensure that the patient is allowed to participate at least equally and the patient should be encouraged to talk. The nurse will need to employ listening and attention-giving skill to gain maximum diversional effect.

Counselling

This may help, particularly with anxieties, problems or conflicts.

Suggestion

In nursing, this usually means to inculcate an idea or thought in another person without him or her realizing that it was not originally his or her own. The person making the suggestion is controlling the other in a very subtle way. Suggestion may in itself have diversional properties. It may direct the person away from unacceptable thoughts and may also bring about desired behaviour in the person in question. Roberts (1971) describes three kinds of suggestion: (i) direct; (ii) semi-direct; and (iii) indirect. Direct suggestion is a disguised form of request, advice or permission, e.g. 'Would you like to come and help me?'; 'It may help if you read this book'. Semi-direct suggestion links the nurse with the person: 'If I were you I would ask the wife to bring your modelling equipment for you'; 'Perhaps we could have a chat'. Indirect suggestion usually points to the required thought or behaviour by projecting it on to a third person, other object or situation, e.g. 'Most of the other patients go to the occupational therapist to see if she can help'.

Suggestion may not be accepted immediately. The seeds of suggestion often grow to bring forth fully developed ideas and thoughts that the person generally believes to be his or her own. This requires time, patience and sometimes repeated suggestion. The nurse, by identifying the patient's needs and motives, will be in a better position to divert his or her attention by using suggestion. Some people are more suggestible than others and the nurse's power to influence other people should be used with care and respect for the other person.

Persuasion

This generally describes a situation in which one person encourages another to change his or her mind or do something against his or her will. Some pressure is exerted to influence the other person in this change. Brown and Murphy (1976) describe persuasion as: '. . .efforts to induce beliefs or actions through argument, pleading or urging'.

The element of pressure suggests that this method of diversion should be carried out only after careful consideration and in the best interests of the patient. Nurses must examine their motives carefully before indulging in this exercise of influence. Some forms of persuasion, such as logical argument and pleading, are acceptable in nursing practice. Others such as threat, lies or deceit are not. Illicit use of persuasion can destroy the patient's confidence in the nurse. It may also cause negative reactions and hostility in the patient if he or she does not want to change and he or she realizes that social pressure is being put upon him or her. Persuasion is best carried out only when absolutely necessary and all else fails in directing the person away from unacceptable thoughts or actions. Rapport with the patient and respect for him or her will enable the nurse to use persuasion without detrimental effect. Tact and a pleasant, sincere manner will also prove an asset. Roberts (1971) suggests the following procedure for persuasion:

1. Agree and approve of aspects the patient believes in or is doing.
2. Build confidence by reassuring.
3. Suggest alternative thoughts or actions.
4. Leave the patient for a short time to think things over.
5. Ask later if the patient has come to a decision.
6. As a last resort, imply disapproval or disinterest in a casual way.

Occupational Therapy

The approach here is the involvement of the patient in physical and/or mental tasks that occupy the person and make demands on his or her attention and concentration. This may involve formal referral to the occupational therapist but nurses are likely to be involved as well. The activities may include work, crafts, hobbies, physical exercise, sport and industrial therapy. Generally, the activity should be compatible with the need for diversion. If thought disorder or emotional problems are present, the form of occupation should reasonably be expected to interfere with these preoccupations. Physical effort can provide an acceptable outlet to aggressive or destructive tendencies.

On occasions, occupational activities restore a person's confidence in himself or herself and his or her abilities, even though sometimes this is only short-lasting. Social activities such as some recreational pursuits (e.g. dances, team sport) encourage the patient to engage in social interaction, thus producing the diversional effect. The following considerations will help in the provision of occupational activities:

1. Identify the patient's diversional need.
2. Determine the interests and abilities of the patient.
3. Assess the effect of the patient's illness and treatment on his or her ability to participate in the tasks.
4. Decide on the occupational pursuit, with the patient.
5. Provide the situation and equipment.
6. Help the patient to carry out activity or participate and facilitate.
7. Evaluate the effectiveness of the activity.

REFLECTIVE ACTIVITIES

1. Write down all the possible reasons (motives) you can think of to explain why you are carrying out this task.
2. From the list of motives produced from Activity 1, decide whether each reason is an example of intrinsic motivation, drive-reduction or operant conditioning.
3. When you want someone else to do something, especially if he or she is likely to be uncooperative or reluctant, attempt to use the method for motivating others described in the text.
4. Plan and carry out a teaching exercise in each of the following situations: (i) a friend who would be prepared to learn a skill; (ii) a junior nurse who does not know how to carry out a particular nursing skill; (iii) a patient who must learn something to promote his or her recovery in hospital or at home.
5. Try writing out some learning outcomes for skills that you carry out every day at work.
6. Next time you meet a patient with chronic pain, try to use some of the methods of diversional technique in addition to the treatment he or she has been prescribed.
7. Next time a patient says that he or she is bored, use the principles for providing occupational activities as described in the text.

SELF-EVALUATION TASKS

Do not read these questions until you are sure you have learned and understood the preceding chapter.

1. Define the following terms: extrinsic motivation; operant conditioning; frustration; teaching.
2. List at least nine situations encountered in nursing that require teaching skill from the nurse.
3. List at least three stages of a 'teaching process', including under each stage those actions that enable the stage to be achieved.
4. List and briefly describe 10 principles for giving feedback when teaching.
5. List at least 10 situations in nursing practice when diversional technique may be useful.
   Check your answers with the text.

CHAPTER 9

Skills for social control

LEARNING OBJECTIVES

You should concentrate on being able to:

1. Define the terms: group; power; leadership; group norm; communication channel; sociogram; sociomatrix; aggression; violence.
2. Give four examples of groups the nurse may have to lead or influence.
3. List 13 possible functions of a leader.
4. List the four stages of a 'leadership process'.
5. List six reasons why people form groups.
6. Draw diagrams to show each of the common communication networks for five-person groups.
7. Draw up a sociogram from the observation of a small group (5–12 persons), marking off the number of times each person spoke to each other person by communication lines.
8. List and describe each of the types of social relationship that may be identified as a sociogram.
9. Assess the contribution from any group member in terms of consistent verbal and non-verbal responses to other group members.
10. List five methods of goal-setting.
11. Identify the type of leadership of a small group in terms of authoritarian, democratic or *laissez-faire* control.
12. Assess a group in terms of Halpin and Croft's 'climates'.
13. List the behaviour of a leader that would facilitate a given group climate.
14. Describe the personality characteristics that will enhance group leadership.
15. List 10 methods of evaluating leadership efficiency.
16 List the types of harm that may be caused to one or both parties when violence has occurred.
17. Describe those situations in nursing practice when aggression and violence are most likely to be met.

18. List seven principles that should be adopted when managing aggression and violence.
19. Describe methods of preventing violence and dealing with aggression.
20. List and briefly describe six general principles that should be followed if one has to intervene physically in violent incidents.
21. Describe the procedure for aftercare following violent incidents.

GROUP LEADERSHIP

There are several occasions when the nurse is compelled to relate to other people, not as individuals but as collections of two or more people. When the nurse relates to one person, the situation can be described as a dyadic interaction. As soon as the nurse relates to two people at one and the same time and each of these participants interacts to achieve the same aim or function, a group has been set up. While accepting the fact that the nurse must work with and deal with many groups in health care settings, two groups are of particular importance in hospital; the ward or departmental nursing team and groups of patients. In a wider context the health care team and the family are also significant groups to the nurse.

As a manager the nurse will need to control the ward nursing team and, in many instances, members of other disciplines, to ensure that the work required from them is carried out. This very often means ensuring that patient care and treatment are carried out with optimum effect. Patients on a ward must be considered as a group in situations such as evacuation in the event of fire, cross-infection and when they are formed into therapeutic groups. Various 'crowds' of people often assemble in the hospital, for example visitors to the ward and patients in waiting areas of hospital departments. Nurses will be all too familiar with this, as it has been a constant feature of hospitals since they were created (Figure 9.1).

In order to engage in group leadership as a skilled action, the nurse must understand fully the meaning of the terms group and leadership. In addition he or she must be able to carry out at least four broad activities: (i) assess each group's characteristics; (ii) define goals; (iii) bring about change with desired effects; and (iv) obtain feedback to estimate group performance.

The Group

At the turn of the century it was fashionable to believe that groups, collections of more than two people, behaved as a unit somewhat unrelated to the individuals making up the group. There arose the idea of collective consciousness or 'group mind' (Le Bon, 1895), which

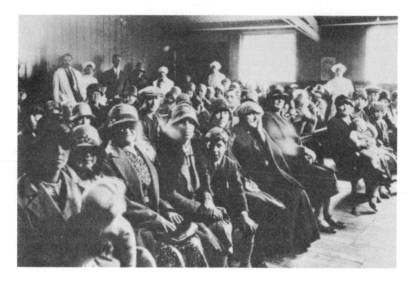

Figure 9.1 Groups have always been an all too familiar aspect of hospital life.

was based on the observation that a person's actions in a crowd differed markedly to his or her behaviour as an individual. There is no evidence to suggest that any psychological or physiological phenomenon exerts any influence over and above the individual person's consciousness (Davis, 1969).

There are, however, two assumptions that will be supported in this discussion and which encourage the nurse to be more reflective about group action. The first is that people co-operate and interact to produce collective action. The second is that group participation brings about behaviour changes in individuals. This latter point is based on the finding that the mere presence of others alters human behaviour. This may promote the efficiency of the person's behaviour in which case it is called social facilitation. Alternatively, the presence of others may have a negative effect on human performance and this is called social inhibition. Zajonc and Sales (1966) suggest that social facilitation occurs because the presence of others is innately arousing and engenders drive (see section in Chapter 7 on motivation). This drive, as it becomes stronger, increases the production of behavioural responses, in particular those readily produced by the individual.

Sherif *et al.* (1961), when studying 12-year-old boys coming together for the first time at summer camp, found that they soon established a sense of co-operation and a group identity, which was a strong source of motivation to individual members. Davis (1969) defines a group as:

'a set of persons by definition or observation among whom there exists a definable or observable set of relations'. A group is a set of mutually interdependent behavioural systems that not only affect each other but respond to exterior influences as well. The notion of a group may seem less mysterious if it is imagined to be composed, first, of a set of individuals and, second, of a collection of interdependent individuals.

Leadership

In any group, one person can become a focus for the attention and behaviour of the other members. This person may be given this position merely because the other members of the group allow or prefer this to occur. This has been described as emergent leadership (Sherif and Sherif, 1953). In relation to nursing teams and patient leadership, the determinant of leadership is often external, being imposed by factors not easily controlled by group members. Thus a leader may have ascribed authority by being appointed by a more powerful agency or pre-existing institutional rules or organizational systems. The ward sister/head nurse is an ascribed leader, the junior nurse and patients having little opportunity to choose or change this leader. This definition of leadership implies an important characteristic of leadership, which is the relationship of a particular person to other group members. The group members respond to the leader in a particular way and this is generally concerned with the degree of influence that this leader exerts in pursuit of particular goals and aims. The leader is a major focus in the attainment of the groups functions. The success or failure of the group hinges on the influence of this leader.

Moloney (1979) summarizes this orientation to nursing leadership by saying that it may be defined as: 'A dynamic, adaptive, interactional, social process of influencing and being influenced by the behaviour of others, and by factors in the situation, in efforts toward goal-setting and goal-achievement within a social system'. She goes on to support the importance of leadership as a nursing social skill by saying: 'The nurse will be either a success or failure in leading others to the extent that she [he] can understand and effectively use this process in fulfilling her [his] leadership responsibilities'. There is also a requirement in exerting leadership to: 'Effect change, to convince the followers to work toward certain goals'.

The ability of the nurse leader will often be measured in terms of the power that he or she has to get other people to do as she requires. The notion of 'power' is closely related to the concept of leadership, playing a significant but not necessarily characteristic part in most 'authority relationships' between groups of people: 'By authority relationship we mean an unequal relationship in which one or several individuals dominate the others and bend them, more or less, to their will' (Duverger, 1972).

It is not uncommon for nurse leaders to have to participate in 'authority relationships' with group members, particularly in an employer/management role. It is important then to identify and acknowledge power relationships when they occur because they influence the effectiveness of nurse leadership and the nature of his or her ascribed relationship to group members.

An interesting point about power relationships is that they might, at the same time, embody antagonistic and integrative facets. Duverger (1972) exemplifies this by reference to Janus the two-faced god. Power relationships in a political sense at the same time attempt to achieve goals for the good of the whole group but, by demanding conformity and compliance, can bring people into antagonistic conflict with each other. This is an important consideration for the nurse who is given authority. In group situations, as a leader, he or she will need to balance those actions that aim to achieve the group aims with those that may cause conflict with group members.

The discussion so far suggests that groups work on the basis of a single leader in every situation. Yet it is possible to have groups that are influenced by two leaders; at one time and by different leaders for different functions (Gillies, 1989). Carter (1953), for instance, found that in one group carrying out six different types of tasks, one person tended to be leader in intellectual activities and another person leader for object manipulation tasks. Attempts to find a single leadership personality have, in fact, been unproductive (Gibb, 1949; Mann, 1959), and the general trend is to accept the fact that the choice of person taking up the leadership position and the success of his or her leadership depends upon the unique combination of personalities, and the structure and function of each individual group (McKeachie and Doyle, 1970).

When assuming leadership it is as well to understand the possible functions that this role entails. These functions are important because the needs of group members will influence the nurse leader's approach. The list below from Kretch *et al.*, (1962) shows the many functions that a leader may serve in a group:

1. Executive – carrying out, bringing action into effect.
2. Planner.
3. Policy-maker – decides rules and course of action.
4. Expert – possessor of knowledge.
5. External group representative – speaks for group.
6. Controller of internal relations.

7. Purveyor of punishment and rewards.
8. Arbitrator and mediator.
9. Exemplar or model, for group members to copy.
10. Substitute for individual responsibility.
11. Ideologist.
12. Father figure.
13. Scapegoat – person to take the blame.

A final point on leadership is that although there is some evidence to suggest that leaders are 'born', it is just as feasible that people can be trained to be 'leaders' (Jack, 1934).

GROUP CONTROL SKILLS

The ability to control a group as a leader will be discussed by considering it as a four-stage process of: (i) analysis; (ii) goal-setting; (iii) execution of influence; and (iv) evaluation of effect. The astute reader will recognize that these stages are comparable with the nursing process stages of: (i) assessment; (ii) planning; (iii) action; and (iv) evaluation. This is because they are both problem-solving processes.

Group Analysis

The discussion of this stage is influenced by the comments of Tannebaum and Schmidt (1958): 'the successful leader . . . accurately understands himself [herself], the individuals and group he [she] is dealing with, and the company and broader social environment in which he [she] operates . . . [and] . . . is able to behave appropriately in the light of these perceptions'.

In order to carry out nursing leadership one should be able to observe **and** assess certain attributes of any given group. The most commonly accepted group phenomena will be discussed here in the belief that greater knowledge will assist the nurse's awareness and analysis of the groups she must control. These are: (i) types of group; (ii) group norms; (iii) communication systems; (iv) group cohesion and morale; and (v) individual contribution.

Types of Group

Two major types of group are the primary group and the secondary group. Primary groups are generally small groups that are characterized by face-to-face interaction of its members. They are generally highly cohesive, i.e. have a strong sense of togetherness and group identity. The ward nursing team is a good example of a primary group. Secondary groups are mostly the opposite of primary groups; they are large, there is little face-to-face contact, no member of the group meets every other member, and there is weak cohesion or ties of common purpose. Crowds or groups such as 'the nursing profession' can be viewed as secondary groups.

Groups may also be distinguished by the functions that they serve for the members of the group. People may join groups for the following reasons:

1. Achievement of particular goals or interests, e.g. nursing team, student group, stamp-collecting society, musical appreciation groups and photography club.
2. Group participation is the only way of achieving aims. Many activities such as group sports cannot be carried out individually, e.g. committees, tug-of-war team, football team. While nursing can be carried out individually, health care is generally carried out in groups because one person is unable to perform all functions alone.
3. Affiliative need. Members may have formed or joined a group simply to be with others, e.g. dinner parties, dances and social clubs. One should always remember that whatever the stated function of any group, some members may participate mainly to meet affiliative needs.
4. To gain prestige. Some groups benefit the members by indicating some status or additional importance of individuals because of some exclusive selection criterion. The elite golf club, Mensa and The House of Lords can be viewed as prestigious groups. Sometimes people undertake various occupations because of the prestige that this group is thought to hold. Many professions attract members in this way.
5. Personal material gain. Some groups are formed so that each member may gain money or commodities. A team of bank robbers, while being considered antisocial, provide an excellent example of such a group.
6. Protection. It has been suggested that the basic instinct for the formation of individuals into groups is to protect the members from danger and harm. Modern examples may include professional or trades unions, military patrols and neighbourhood watch schemes.

Jennings (1950) suggested a simpler dichotomy of group type according to the requirements of group members. Groups in which members are interested in the goals of the group he termed **socio**

groups and those in which members are mainly attracted to other members he called **psyche groups**.

Another way of classifying groups has special reference to nursing because it demonstrates the different forms of helping groups (Brown, 1986). The types that have been described include:

1. Individual assessment groups.
2. Individual support and maintenance groups.
3. Individual change groups.
4. Education, information and training groups.
5. Group change and support groups.

Group Norms

Norms are described as 'expected modes of behaviour and beliefs that are established either formally or informally by the group . . . norms guide behaviour and facilitate interaction by specifying the kinds of reactions expected or acceptable in a particular situation' (Jones and Gerard, 1967). The nurse leader will need to identify the standards, rules and expectations of the group in question. Some will be defined by the group itself, others by a previous leader and yet others by external agents or higher authorities. Occasionally, the norms that the group sets may be in conflict with the requirements of the individual. Various studies (Yablonsky, 1962; Sherif, 1936) describe how group norms easily emerge and how group members will conform to them even at risk of severe external penalties.

Communication Systems

The communication that exists within a group may be analysed in terms of: (i) the communication channels available; (ii) the pattern of communication between members; and (iii) the type of contribution made by each member's communicative act. McKeachie and Doyle (1970) say that if one member of a group ever communicates with another member, a communication channel exists between them. Implicit in this assertion is the fact that where a communication channel exists the persons are allowed to communicate. When obstacles prevent various members communicating with each other, particular communication networks may be observed (Bavelas, 1950). Communication networks are of importance to the nurse leader because they demonstrate the variety of possible communicative group structures and point to the effects of limiting the possibility of communication between some group members. If these communication channels are drawn in the form of graphs, five common types of five-person communication networks can be demonstrated (Figure 9.2).

The chain indicates linear exchange of information, each person having to receive information from one person and pass it on to only one different individual. Once the chain is broken the information flow stops.

The wheel indicates a situation in which only one person is able to communicate with every member, each other member communicating only with him or her. It is fairly easy to conceive of situations in which group members only communicate with a leader but not with each other for competitive or jealous reasons.

The circle allows communication with only two other people. The individual depends on these two others to give and pass on information to other group members. This is still fairly restrictive but less likely to fail than the chain.

The Y network described by Leavitt (1951) is a modification of the wheel but it also incorporates the features of a small chain for three of the group members.

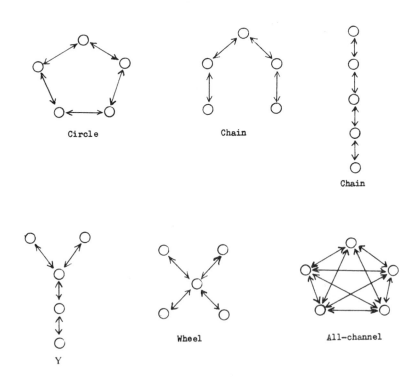

Figure 9.2 Common five-person communication networks. Source: adapted from McKeachie and Doyle (1970).

All-channel communication is the final five-person communication network. Here each member is free to communicate with each other member.

When assessing communication networks, one needs to decide whether the communication channel is one-way or two-way. A one-way channel points to the individual who receives information from another. If he is allowed to reciprocate by giving information to the sender as well, a two-way channel is set up. Figure 9.3 shows how a group of students and the teacher may be described in graphical terms using one- and two-way communication lines. The group learning setting is easily detectable and the method of leadership can also be inferred from a diagram of the communication network. The nurse can draw up communication networks such as these by noting, as a result of observation, who is allowed to approach whom, and whether the recipient pays any attention to the sender of information. In controlled situations, and sometimes in everyday settings, one can observe a

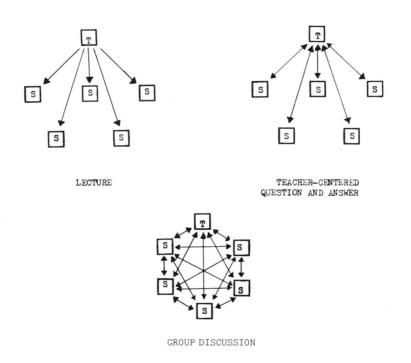

LECTURE

TEACHER–CENTERED
QUESTION AND ANSWER

GROUP DISCUSSION

Figure 9.3 Teacher–student interaction patterns T = teacher; S = student. Source: adapted from McKeachie and Doyle (1970).

group for short periods throughout a day, noting the frequency with which each person communicates with another, drawing a line between each of the two members concerned and the direction of the message. As these lines build up, a pattern can emerge as shown in Figure 9.4 and what is known as a sociogram is produced.

In large groups of eight or more, a simpler alternative is sometimes to draw up a sociomatrix (Davis, 1969), in which a tick can be placed in each box when pairs receive or send information. The rows are used to mark out the sender and columns the receiver. In Figure 9.5, Brown has communicated with Crow. In Figure 9.6 a full matrix is represented. Sociograms and sociomatrices help the nurse leader to represent and analyse the structure of the group. An additional form of sociometry analyses group structure by assessing each individual member's preferences for other group members (Moreno, 1943). Each member is asked in some anonymous form to indicate whom he or she would prefer to have as a partner in several activities. These preferences are then drawn up in the form of a sociogram (Figure 9.7).

Various relationships or roles may be identified in these sociograms. (Lee, 1976) describes seven types of social relationship, which are shown in Figure 9.7.

1. The star, the most popular student, marked S.
2. The reciprocated or mutual pair. Indicates choice of friendships that are mutual, e.g. M and M.

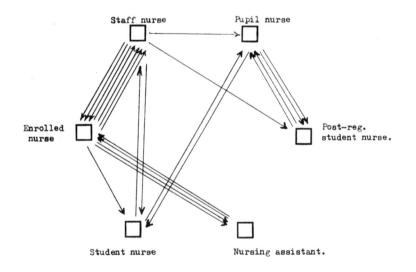

Figure 9.4 Analysis of amount of communication between group members of a ward team over a certain time period.

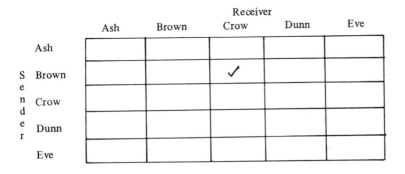

Figure 9.5 Entry on sociomatrix indicating Brown's communication to Crow.

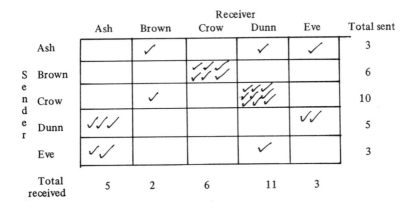

Figure 9.6 Full sociomatrix showing communications between members of a five-person group over a certain time period.

3. Chain structures. The reciprocal choices marked by members, marked C, show this form of relationship.
4. The triangle shows a clique within the group, in this case a triad marked T.
5. The rejectee is the person rejected by others while not being chosen by anybody at all, labelled R.
6. The neglectee is a person not rejected by anyone but not chosen either. He or she is ignored, labelled N.
7. The isolate is a person who makes and receives no choices, labelled I.

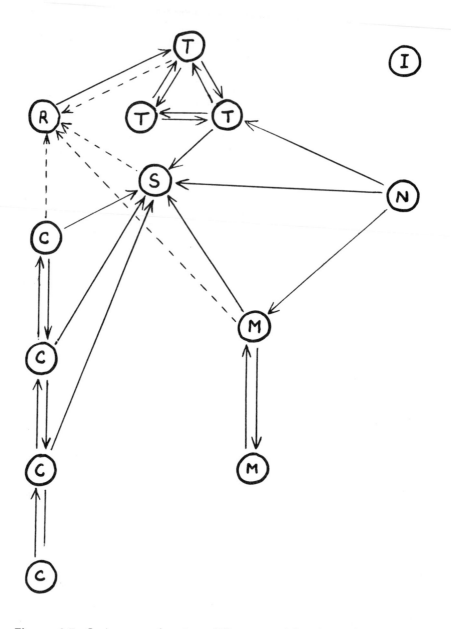

Figure 9.7 Sociogram showing different social relationships and constructed from stated preferences: —— = positive choices; ---- = negative choices; arrows show direction of choice.

Assessing Individual Contributions

Each individual can be assessed as has already been demonstrated, simply on the number of messages he or she sends and receives. Some members may then be seen as highly vocal or noisy participants; these may be the ones who exert influence over the actions of the other group members. They may have power, which causes problems if they compete with ascribed leaders or have detrimental effects on leadership ability. Some members produce many ideas or may be experts on the task in question. Others may facilitate problem-solving or decision-making. Quiet individuals are rarely non-participative and one must assess them by observing non-verbal cues. Some quiet people have a great influence over group proceedings by their selective and effective use of non-verbal communication. While this may present a confusing picture, there are methods available to assess the nature of individual contributions. Perhaps the most popular is that described by Bales (1950) who proposes assessment of each individual's contribution on the basis of the response checklist shown in Figure 9.8. As can be seen, one can assess whether a person is mainly concerned with positive and negative aspects of orientation, evaluation, control, decision-making, tension, management or integration.

Goal-setting

Goal-setting can involve the following procedures:

1. Defining group goals or receiving goals or orders from external authority.
2. Assessing the needs of group members.
3. Writing objectives.
4. Communication of goals to all group members and external entities.
5. Balance-sheet analysis (see Chapter 7).

The Execution of Influence

It has been suggested that leadership involves the control of group members to bring about change. Leadership can thus cause tension in group members, as well as in the organizations and institutions of which the group are a part. Several authors suggest that this is in many respects inevitable if the leader is to be successful: 'Dynamic leaders are expected to cause ripples . . . without ripples, even change is unlikely to occur' (Leininger, 1974); 'A leader must lead . . . must rock the boat . . . must disturb people . . . must initiate change . . . must take risks . . . take responsibility for both his or her failures and successes' (Halpin, 1965).

	1	Shows solidarity, raises other's status, gives help, reward.	f
A	2	Shows tension release, jokes, laughs, shows satisfaction.	e
	3	Agrees, shows passive acceptance, understands, concurs, complies.	d
	4	Gives suggestion, direction, implying autonomy for others.	c
B	5	Gives opinion, evaluation, analysis, expresses feelings, wishes.	b
	6	Gives orientation, information, repeats, clarifies, confirms.	a
	7	Asks for orientation, information, repetition, confirmation.	a
C	8	Asks for opinion, evaluation, analysis, expression of feeling.	b
	9	Asks for suggestion, direction, possible ways of action.	c
	10	Disagrees, shows passive rejection, formality, witholds help.	d
D	11	Shows tension, asks for help, withdraws out of field.	e
	12	Shows antagonism, deflates others status, defends or asserts self.	f

Key:
A = positive reactions   a = Problem of communication or orientation
B = attempted answers   b = Problems of evaluation
                                 c = Problems of control
C = questions   d = Problems of decision
                                 e = Problems of tension reduction
D = negative reactions   f = Problems of reintegration

Figure 9.8 Bale's interaction categories.

However, one should qualify this by saying that leaders should minimize the negative or destructive effects of their control. One must bear in mind that the execution of influence requires complex skill development given that a firm insistence that one's own view is the only correct one and that it should be adopted by all the others in the group, is unlikely to be helpful. Similarly, a tendency to take control and dominate a group is likely to be unproductive in the long run (Nichols and Jenkinson, 1991). The execution of influence will be discussed under three headings: (i) group climate; (ii) personality of the leader; and (iii) directive behaviour.

Group Climate

The leader's action can influence the group's climate or attitudes. One of the earliest pairs of studies associated with this aspect were undertaken by White and Lippitt (1960) and Lewin (1947). They describe three types of leadership style producing a particular orientation in the group members affected:

Authoritarian style (autocratic)

Policy is determined by the leader, who also dictates action and communication structure. The leader is dominant, dogmatic, using positive acts of command, direction, reinforcement and information-giving to encourage members to co-operate with his or her wishes. He or she tends to remain aloof from group participation and to criticize group members' personalities.

Democratic style (participative or supportive leadership)

This style encourages the group members to participate in the decision-making process. The leader helps them to do this while participating in group activities. White and Lippitt found this sort of leader was 'objective' or 'fact-minded' in his or her praise or criticism. These groups tend to be activity orientated, outlining a series of steps to meet the required goal. The members have freedom to choose whom they work with and task allocation is decided by the group as a whole.

Laissez-faire style (free rein)

The group members are allowed complete freedom with a minimum of leader participation. The group members can make decisions indepen-dently of the leader and set whatever goals they think fit. The leader becomes a resource, providing information and materials only when asked and does not join in group activities, there generally being no attempt to appraise or regulate the course of events. Often group members enjoy this style of control initially but later become tense, confused and dissatisfied with the lack of leadership (Moloney, 1979). It has been suggested as a result of the work of White and Lippitt (1960) that democratic group members are more productive than either of the other two group types and are more interested and involved in the group activities. Authoritarian leadership often brings about aggressive behaviour in group members, while *laissez-faire* group members tend to waste a lot of time in non-purposeful activity.

Climate Facilitation

When setting the climate of group organization, it is possible to consider six types of climate described from the work of Halpin and Croft (1963), who studied the organizational structure of elementary schools. These, adapted from Moloney (1979), are:

1. The **open** climate. This is characterized by high morale, members working well together, leader facilitation, high motivation, pride in organization, active leadership, and the leader not being aloof.
2. The **autonomous** climate. This is characterized by freedom, a tendency to meet social needs, members working well together, with a high morale, where the leader is aloof, not 'pushy' but works hard.
3. The **controlled** climate. This is characterized by the need for achievement rather than social needs, with a hard-working approach, a high morale, few policies and procedures, impersonal relationships, task orientation, with the leader dominating and directive and very little leadership delegation.
4. The **familiar** climate. This is characterized by friendliness, social need, motivation, little task achievement, average morale and satisfaction, the leader is neither aloof nor impersonal but considerate. Full work capacity is not achieved.
5. The **paternal** climate. This is characterized by ineffective leader control, members split into factions (cliques), low morale, dissatisfaction of group members, with the task and social needs unmet, the leader intrusive, poor motivation, and the leader considerate for selfish reasons.
6. The **closed** climate. This is characterized by minimal group satisfaction, little co-operation or joint action, with the leader being aloof, impersonal, inconsiderate, ungenuine and ineffective in leadership ability.

Leadership action will be determined by the type of group climate required and the needs of the group in question, i.e. whether they are formed to meet task or social goals. Several skills such as listening, counselling, motivation, teaching, explanation, reassurance and communication skills will need to be employed selectively to achieve the climate required to bring about the required changes.

Personality/Self Concept of the Leader

The nurse leader will find that certain behavioural tendencies that are characteristic of his or her personality will make it difficult for her to take certain courses of action while facilitating others. The nurse who has high affiliative need may be reluctant to risk upsetting her followers, thus possibly making it difficult for her to communicate her requirements or give commands.

A newly acquired leadership role will not always fit the nurse's personality and B. Stevens (1975) suggests that the nurse must recognize the discrepancies and change the focus of his or her role. This involves the ability to carry out self-appraisal, capitalize on or minimize appropriate personality traits and to recognize areas for training and development. A behaviourist approach would probably suggest that the nurse can learn coping strategies or responses to the particular problems that he or she meets. There is evidence to suggest that leaders can be trained to make responses for particular situations (Jack, 1934; Hastorf, 1965; Gibb, 1969; Bavelas *et al.* 1965).

What then can we suggest as useful characteristic behaviours of good leaders? Bales (1950) found that two types of leader emerge in unstructured groups: (i) one who guides the discussion and has the best ideas; (ii) the other who is liked best by group members, adopts tension-releasing behaviour and concerns himself or herself with maintaining group unity. Halpin and Winer (1957) also discovered two similar dimensions. The first was the amount of **consideration** for group members' ideas, attitudes and feelings. This dimension consisted of positive and negative roles, at one end the leader being tolerant and supportive, at the other end intolerant and unsupportive. The second dimension suggested is **initiating structure**, the ability of the leader to plan and direct group activity. This would involve motivational ability. Democratic groups are high in leader 'considera-tion' and 'initiating ability' and as they are considered more effective than authoritarian and *laissez-faire* groups, one can infer that they are successful leadership behaviours.

One could ask whether a successful leader should be friendly with group members and whether this determines successful leadership. Evidence from Hollander and Webb (1955) suggests that friendship is not the chief determinant of good leadership, yet consideration for others is. It appears then that people do not necessarily need or want friendly relations with leaders. The group task will also dictate who will be leader. Carter (1953) found that one person in a group tended to emerge as leader for intellectual tasks and another person for object manipulation tasks. This suggests that it may be necessary for some leaders to step down from their role if they are not the best person to lead the task in hand, reassuming leadership once the task is completed.

An important determinant of leadership success concerns the situational variations that groups are subject to. Fiedler (1974) suggests that this variation is associated mainly with 'situational control'. This is a measure of the amount of control and influence the person

believes that he or she has over group activity. According to Fiedler
(1974) one can create a situation in which the members have high
situational control by: (i) adopting a positive and trusting relationship
between leader and group; (ii) structuring the task so that members
know what to do; and (iii) rewarding and punishing members.

The leader's influence on the group climate is important because the
functioning of the group can be determined by this and the group
performance may subsequently be either creative, intermediate, or
destructive in its outcome (Dainow and Bailey, 1988).

Directive Behaviour

The importance of motivational and reinforcement skills must be
highlighted at this point, being appropriate methods of encouraging
others to co-operate with the leader's requirements. Other actions,
however, which are more persuasive, must also be used. On occasions,
leaders in institutions must exercise power over others to ensure that
they comply. An interesting piece of research by Falbo and Peplau
(1980) lists commonly used strategies that people used to 'get their
own way' when disagreement occurred in interpersonal transactions
(Table 9.1).

One can add to this section on direct control by listing the
intellectual and personal qualities described in *Leadership in Nursing*
(Moloney, 1979). These qualities of the nurse leader point to several
effective leadership actions that may be adopted (Table 9.2).

Table 9.1 How People control Decision-making When Disagreement Occurs

Strategy	Example
1. Ask	'I ask him or her to do what I want.'
2. Act independently	'We do our own thing. I just do it by myself.'
3. Bargain	'We usually negotiate something agreeable to both of us.'
4. Act negatively	'I pout or threaten to cry if I don't get my own way.'
5. Persist	'I remind him or her of what I want until he or she gives in.'
6. Persuade	'I persuade him or her my way is right.'
7. Act positively	'I smile a lot, and am especially affectionate.'
8. Reason	'I reason with him or her. I argue logically.'
9. State importance	'I tell him or her how important it is to me.'
10. Suggest	'I drop hints, make suggestions.'
11. Talk it out	'We discuss our needs and differences.'
12. State my goals	'I tell him or her what I want.'
13. Withdrawal	'I clam up.'

Source: Falbo and Peplau, 1980.

Table 9.2   Qualities of Leadership

Intellectual Qualities	*Personal Qualities*
1. Use one's intelligence	1. Maintain sound health and mental and physical vigour
2. Analyse, interpret accurately	2. Be personally attractive, vivacious and enthusiastic
3. Organize, synthesize	3. Endure hard work, long hours, stress and fatigue
4. Make decisions	4. Be well-dressed, neat and poised
5. Use sound judgment	5. Control gestures, mannerisms, tone and behaviour
6. Weigh alternatives	6. Relate well to others
7. Sort out relevant from irrelevant	7. Be creative
8. Motivate and influence others	8. Develop and use a sense of humour
9. Set realistic goals	9. Exercise self-control and self-discipline
10. Teach and transmit knowledge	10. Respect and affirm self and others
11. Be perceptive and insightful	11. Convey trust, openness and sincerity
12. Be realistic and authentic	12. Communicate well with various public agencies
13. Use theories of leadership	13. Uphold decisions and do not vacillate
14. Strong achievement drive	14. Tolerate a high level of frustration
	15. Be uniquely individual

Source: Moloney, 1979.

Evaluation of Leadership Efficiency

The successful nurse leader will need constantly to assess the effect of his or her actions on the group as a whole as well as on individual group members, and will need to adopt strategies to receive feedback. Several suggestions for receiving feedback from groups, many of which have already been mentioned in this text, are given below:

- observation;
- listening;
- counselling;
- participation in group activity;
- open-door policy/approachability;
- suggestion box;
- group discussion, e.g. meetings;
- measurement of productivity;
- evaluation of task completion;
- questioning, using interview and questionnaire
- improvement meetings (quality circles);
- nominal group evaluation.

DEALING WITH VIOLENCE AND AGGRESSION

The terms aggression and violence are used here to describe two closely related but different situations. Aggression describes a situation in which a person displays an emotion that is potentially destructive. In some countries, this comes within the legal definition of assault (Keltner *et al.*, 1991) It is generally directed towards one object or person at any one time and is an action or gesture that suggests that an act of violence is likely to occur. Violence, on the other hand, describes a situation in which one person exercises physical force so as to inflict injury or damage to persons or property.

Dealing with aggression and violence is described here as a social skill because it involves the nurse and patient in interpersonal transaction and requires the nurse to be trained to take decisions and controlled action in pursuit of particular goals. Nurses are required to act in the best interests of the patient and themselves, adopting guidelines and procedures that are most likely to alleviate this unique situation. Such situations are unusual because they are likely to be emotionally charged, engendering fear in one or both of the participants. This sudden increase of emotional energy causes the greatest of difficulties for the nurse. The danger is that he or she is likely to react spontaneously, irrationally and excessively in response to his or her fear. Skilled action would involve appropriate knowledge, empathic understanding of the patient and the use of 'tried and trusted' acceptable methods to prevent injury to either party during the incident. All of this must be carried out in a controlled manner, which means that the nurse must learn and practise the art of dealing with these difficult social situations. This relates in part to Chapter 6 where reassurance was discussed as a skill for dealing with anxiety or fear in patients.

What Harm May Be Done?

It has already been suggested that injury may occur to one or both of the persons involved. Sometimes the person may injure himself by self-mutilation rather than harm another person. It has also been suggested that property may be damaged and, while this is an important consideration when dealing with violent persons, it should never take priority over human injury. In addition to physical damage, aggression as well as violence may cause harm to another person's emotional stability and this may affect the nurse who is the focus of the aggression or a passive observer. The nurse may become anxious or insecure, while other patients and staff may become anxious or lose confidence in the nurse who is the object of aggression. Finally, damage can obviously occur to the rapport between the nurse and the aggressive person, indeed rapport may be completely destroyed.

When are Aggression and Violence likely to occur?

The simple answer to this is to assume always and often at the most unexpected times. It is not, however, productive to be always on one's guard for aggressive and violent outbursts and certain situations indicate aggression and violence more often than others. They are briefly listed below as a guide, always bearing in mind that one should never expect that violence will occur but only accept the possibility of its occurrence.

1. Accident and Emergency Department (DHSS, 1976).
2. Where patients are intoxicated by drugs or alcohol (DHSS, 1976).
3. Patients who are confused.
4. Patients who are hypoglycaemic.
5. Patients after grand mal epileptic seizure.
6. Patients during temporal lobe epileptic seizure.
7. Patients who are febrile.
8. Patients with severe electrolyte imbalance (i.e. uraemia).
9. Patients who are severely hallucinated.
10. Patients who are severely deluded.
11. Patients who are physically overactive (e.g. mania).
12. Patients who are severely brain damaged or severely mentally handicapped.
13. Psychological disturbance during pregnancy.
14. Where persons are suspected of carrying offensive weapons (DHSS, 1976).
15. Shortly after aggressive and violent incidents from others not involved in original incident.
16. Where persons experience severe frustration, e.g. compulsory hospital detention, physical disability, long wait in waiting rooms.
17. Where there is overcrowding (DHSS, 1976).
18. Persons who have recently or are undergoing extreme stress.
19. Where there is custodial care and few therapeutic activities (DHSS, 1976).
20. Any person acting in a strange manner and who is not known to the nurse.
21. People with a recent history of violence.

Management of Aggression and Violence

Where aggression and violence occur, the nurse will find it necessary to interact with the aggressive person in several ways in order to prevent or minimize the harm that may be done. When applying the principles associated with this social skill the nurse should aim to achieve the following:

1. Minimize the harmful effects with a minimum amount of antagonism or physical intervention.
2. Protect self, the patient and others from physical injury.
3. Maintain the dignity and self-respect of the aggressive/violent patient as much as possible.
4. Preserve as much rapport between self and the patient during and after the incident. Maintain a positive relationship.
5. Ensure that one does not lose control over one's actions.
6. Maintain communication with others not initially involved in the incident. Enlist help from as many people as possible and report all incidents to others.
7. Use the situation as an opportunity for learning by both the patient and nurse involved.

The management of violence may be examined in three stages: (i) prevention; (ii) incident management; and (iii) aftercare. Dealing with aggression is covered by the section on preventing violence and only a few comments specific to dealing with aggression will be made.

Prevention of Violence and Dealing with Aggression

There is still much reluctance to give practical guidance on the prevention and management of violence and, as such, the subject is still neglected in education programmes. Practical advice is sparse and sometimes dated (DHSS, 1976; South East Thames Regional Health Authority, 1980; Goldman, 1992). It is commonly agreed, however, that by far the best way of dealing with violence is prevention. Three basic approaches can be adopted to achieve this: (i) get to know the patient well; (ii) achieve a close relationship; and (iii) observe for signs of impending violence. Knowledge of the patient as a person, his or her illness, social background and history will help the nurse to understand the reasons for the patient's aggression. Knowledge of the patient also enables the nurse to make predictions as to how he or she may behave or what effective action the nurse could take. Many a nurse has begun to calm an aggressive patient by asking him about his favourite hobby or what the latest football result is. While this will never solve the problem on its own, it can help to break the tension in a difficult situation. The achievement of rapport by the nurse or at least one member of staff can help in situations of aggression on the assumption that the aggressive person is less likely to harm someone he is close to and may also be more susceptible to the help and intervention of this person. If one is to achieve a close relationship then it is clear that some of the counselling skills (Chapter 7) such as genuineness, respect, empathic understanding and immediacy can be employed to some advantage in this situation.

Observations for signs of aggression and impending violence will assist in preventing violence by providing enough time to take simple action that may avert a crisis. The nurse may observe restlessness, bizarre behaviour, threats, facial expressions or gestures that indicate anger. He or she may notice various antagonistic features such as overcrowding, excessive heat and persons interfering, manipulating or taunting the patient. When such observations are made they are useless if they are not acted upon and reported to colleagues. Observation will also lead to an assessment of the likelihood of violence. In some situations violence appears imminent – likely to occur at any second. In other situations, one can see that the state of affairs may lead to violence in the next few hours. Occasionally, there is no warning of violence at all. Clearly these three situations warrant different courses of action. It would be a waste of time to adopt a counselling approach if a person had his or her fist clenched and was ready to strike the nurse.

Several additional actions can be taken to help prevent violence. When nurses meet aggression they should avoid reacting aggressively themselves. Meeting aggression with aggression tends to make things worse because a win-or-lose situation is set up and this tends to perpetuate the problem until a result one way or the other is achieved. Winning and losing are not aims of this social skill. The nurse should also avoid subconscious attempts to threaten the patient at this stage. Where a person insults the nurse or shouts at him or her, he or she should try to accept this with good grace but without being flippant or condescending. The nurse should not laugh or make jokes inappropriately. He or she should not ignore aggression, nor encourage it, for both reactions may make it worse. When a patient is aggressive to gain attention, one should give attention that does not reinforce aggressive behaviour. Ignoring attention-seeking behaviour may only serve to make the person exaggerate the unacceptable behaviour. Attention to his or her own non-verbal behaviour will also help the nurse to cope with aggression and prevent violence. The nurse should try to control any display of fear and should appear calm and in control (Perko and Kriegh, 1988). The nurse should adopt a soothing quiet tone of voice and shouting should only be used to issue a command that may stop a violent person by warning this person or others, and this should have an effect by causing surprise.

When a person gives some indication that he or she is about to be violent, skills of questioning and reassurance should be employed. Ask the patient why he or she is behaving that way and what you can do to help him or her. Explanation may be necessary and counselling also, if time allows. If a patient is about to be violent one can attempt, very gently, to move him or her away from other people or hazards by the use of suggestion or diversional technique but **not** physical contact. When removing the violent patient from others nurses should be careful not to leave themselves alone and expose herself to needless danger or helplessness. Other actions such as maintaining adequate temperature, ventilation and minimizing overcrowding and stress will help to prevent violence. Nurses should minimize unnecessary rules and needless restrictions that would serve to frustrate the patient. Nurses should listen to the patient's fears, frustrations and anxieties, providing sufficient time to allow him or her to express them. Finally, diversional techniques (see Chapter 8) may be employed to redirect the patient's thoughts and excess energies towards acceptable outlets.

Incident Management

When a person becomes violent, one must first assess the type of action to be taken. The first consideration that will determine what action should be taken is whether the violence is directed towards the nurse or other people. Where the nurse is being attacked he or she will take protective action, to ensure that he or she is not injured. Nurses have the same right as any other citizen to restrain the attacker or protect themselves from injury. The Department of Health circular HC (76) 11 describes the situation clearly:

> In law, the general position is that a patient may be restrained or a nurse or other person may protect himself [herself], only with such degree of force as is necessary and reasonable in the circumstances. The more serious the danger the greater the degree of force that may be used to avoid such danger and *vice versa*. Active intervention need not be confined to the person who is threatened by the patient; another person who is not threatened may come to the assistance of the person who is threatened. If it is evident that a violent patient is about to strike somebody he [she] may be restrained before the blow has actually been struck.
>
> *DHSS, 1976*

When other persons or objects are the focus of the violence, the nursing action takes the form of intervention. This must be achieved with as little risk to the nurse as possible. Where persons are likely to be harmed, one may have to take immediate action. Where the violent person is harming himself or herself, this will also demand rapid intervention. Damage to property should not necessitate immediate intervention and at no time should the nurse risk injury to herself or others to prevent damage to property. The person is better left and onlookers evacuated until additional help arrives.

It is tempting at this point to give explicit instructions on how to protect oneself and physically intervene in several situations that may be encountered. Notwithstanding the fact that space does not allow for this in this text, it is folly to give instruction that is likely to be inconsistent with guidelines issued by the administrative body in each local situation. The nurse is therefore strongly advised to read the local guidelines and procedure for dealing with aggression and violent incidents. She must also adhere to them regardless of what is written in this or other texts on the subject. Each move to a different area will mean that the nurse must read and abide by the local procedure. A word of warning is necessary, however, and it is that many guidelines describe what not to do and often circumvent description of what one can do. A good example of positive practical action that can be taken is provided by the booklet *'Guidelines for the Nursing Management of Violence'* (South East Thames Regional Health Authority, 1980). Wherever possible, the learner should encourage his or her teachers to explain in precise terms how one would deal with violent incidents in practical and realistic terms.

Several general principles may be followed when having to intervene physically in violent incidents:

1. Summon as many qualified helpers as possible. Do not approach patients alone unless it is absolutely vital. Learn the local procedure for raising the alarm. Ask other patients to raise the alarm if necessary.
2. Always protect oneself from harm. An injured or unconscious nurse is no good to anybody during the incident. The nurse should never be so cautious or afraid about taking defensive action, because of supposed legal repercussions, that she exposes herself to needless injury.
3. Talk to the patient all the time, even if he or she does not answer. Maintain respect for the patient. Explain what you are doing and your motives when to do so would be helpful.
4. Where physical restraint is necessary, use it as a last resort. Lower the patient to the floor and immobilize him or her by applying pressure to limbs close to joints. Avoid applying pressure directly to bare skin. Ensure clothing cushions the pressure. Do not apply pressure to throat, abdomen or chest.
5. Never kick or strike a blow unless it is the **only** way of protecting oneself from serious injury.
6. Remove jewellery, spectacles, pens and other articles that may cause injury. This should be done where intervention is expected but not in situations of personal attack.

Two examples are given below of procedures that are practical, direct and explicit. They are given here to serve as examples of the sort of knowledge and instruction required if nurses are to be safe, efficient practitioners of this social skill. The reader must remember not to adopt these procedures if they conflict with local policy. The following two examples given are from '*Guidelines for the Nursing Management of Violence*' (South East Thames Regional Health Authority, 1980).

1. Dealing with a personal attack. If you are alone and a patient is violent towards you, another patient or himself (or herself), this will necessitate your immediate action, at least until help arrives. Your aim will be to immobilize the patient either by pressing him or her face forward against a wall, or, preferably, by holding him face downwards on the floor. Do the basic drill: i.e. shout to the patient to stop, call for assistance and sound the alarm bell where possible. If this fails:
   (a) Stay close to the patient;
   (b) Grasp his or her arms at elbow level and pull him or her towards you;
   (c) Quickly change your grip and encircle him or her with your arms;
   (d) Continue pulling him towards you; Then:

Either:	Or:
Quickly get behind the patient push him or her towards a nearby wall	Move to one side. Place nearest leg behind the patient
Retain your grip, lean on him	Keep your foot firmly on the ground
Press him or her to the wall	Push the patient over your leg.
	Lower patient and yourself to the floor.
	Quickly turn the patient onto his or her face.
	Immobilize by laying across his or her trunk.

The above drill, if carried out speedily and efficiently, will enable you to deal with most personal attacks.

2. Hair and tie pulling (Figure 9.9) can be resolved as follows:
   (a) Grasp patient's wrists, pulling hands towards you – hang on;
   (b) Do not attempt to pull away;
   (c) Call for help;
   (d) Shout to the patient to let go.
   If it becomes apparent that the patient will not let go, then, as a last resort, hair or tie may have to be cut. Before this is attempted the patient must be effectively immobilized.

The interested reader is advised to obtain a copy of this booklet

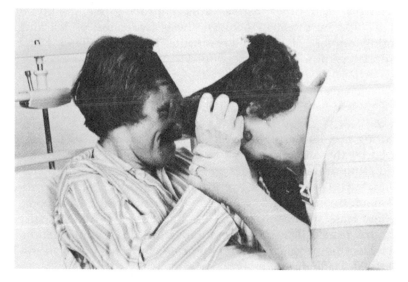

Figure 9.9 Grasp the patient's wrists and pull yourself close – watch his head.

(South East Thames Regional Health Authority, 1980) for information on the possible responses to a variety of other situations. A film has also been made, which demonstrates the procedures described.

Aftercare

Immediately after the incident the nurse and those involved should write a report, on a prescribed report form if necessary. The nurse should also arrange for a full medical examination to ensure that the patient has not been injured. After the incident has passed it is important to do two things. The first is to examine the situation closely so that the people involved, both patient and nurse, may learn from the experience. This can be carried out in the context of a group discussion, which should preferably include the patient and by counselling and explanation from experienced staff. This is an ideal opportunity for reflection, particularly self-reflection. The nurse should aim to improve his or her own skill on the basis of the experience of each violent incident so that he or she will manage future situations with more confidence and efficiency. In addition, he or she should endeavour to help the patient explore the motives for his or her violent behaviour and alternative courses of action that can be taken in future. The second important part of 'aftercare' is the restoration of a positive, useful relationship between the nurse and the patient (and perhaps others involved as well). The nurse will attempt to re-establish the rapport he or she had with the patient before the incident. On some occasions, the nurse and patient may grow to understand each other better, thus improving the quality of the relationship. In order to achieve these two aims of learning and restoring rapport, it should be obvious that counselling will be an appropriate skill for the nurse to use in the long term.

REFLECTIVE ACTIVITIES

1. During a quiet period at work make observations on the methods used by the nurse in charge to lead the nursing team. Also assess the communication channels, leadership style and attitude climate.
2. Draw up a sociogram of a group that you are able to observe. Examples could include a group of patients in the day room, your fellow class members during a coffee break or free period and a theatre team during an operation. Draw in communication lines between the people who communicate with each other on the basis of notes made during a 5-min. period. Make sure this task does not interfere with your duties.
3. The first time you are allowed to lead a group of fellow nurses for any reason and for an appreciable amount of time, make notes on the difficulties and surprises that you experience when attempting to get other people to do what you want.
4. During the observation of a small group, make notes on the contribution of each member to the group activity.
5. Each time you are involved in an aggressive or violent outburst on the ward as an observer or as the recipient of aggression or violence, assess the following at the earliest opportunity you have to consider the situation: (i) the warning signs; (ii) the possible or actual causes; (iii) how much your reactions helped or caused problems; (iv) the effects on you, the patient and your relationship; (v) what action was taken after the incident to help the violent person and other people involved.
6. Ask a friend to sit in a chair and grab your hair or tie as you lean over him or her. Use the procedure described in the procedure 'hair and tie pulling' described in the section on aggressive and violence.

SELF-EVALUATION TASKS

Do not read these questions until you are sure you have learned and understood the preceding chapter.

1. Define the terms: leadership; power; communication channel; sociogram; violence.
2. Give four examples of groups that the nurse may have to lead or control.
3. List the four stages of a leadership process.
4. List and describe each of the social relationships that may be identified on a sociogram.
5. List five methods of goal-setting.
6. Describe the personality characteristics that will enhance group leadership.
7. List the types of harm that may be caused to one or both parties when violence has occurred.
8. List and briefly describe six general principles that should be followed if one has to intervene physically in violent incidents.

Check your answers with the text.

CHAPTER 10

A model for social skills learning

It is now possible to conclude by reviewing the skills described in the preceding chapters with a view to providing a model that will help the learner to decide the most suitable sequence of skill learning. In suggesting a model that summarizes skills and provides a learning plan, one must come to terms with the possible differences between the social skills. The most fundamental differences that may occur will result from varying levels of complexity. It may be obvious, after reading this text, that a skill such as counselling is a more complex activity than a skill such as listening. These two skills also demonstrate the fact that some social skills act as sub-skills to other social skills. Listening, for instance, is one of the many skills that must be mastered in order to become proficient as a counsellor. The complex social skills may therefore differ in the number of simpler skills that they encompass. Knowledge and experience of sub-skills will also contribute to the acquisition of more complex associated skills. By identifying skill levels according to increasing complexity and the inter-relationships between skills, one can generate a hierarchy of social skills that can serve as a heuristic tool or 'rule of thumb guide' to social skill learning in nursing practice. A model in the form of a social skills tree is given in Figure 10.1.

By looking at this tree you may notice some other differences between the social skills described in this book. One is that skills vary in the amount of opportunity to practise them in everyday living. This has important implications for social skills teaching. Some skills such as conversation may be experienced readily in everyday life and the nursing practitioner may be able to draw on his or her past experiences and have more opportunity to practise the skill. Conversely, a skill such as interviewing is relatively unusual in everyday life and previous experience may be totally lacking. Learning will thus depend on the number of interviews that occur in daily work or the number that can be simulated for learning purposes. One may also notice that skills vary in the amount of social involvement between nurse and patient. Some skills, such as balance-sheet analysis and writing personal objectives, do not necessarily rely on any social

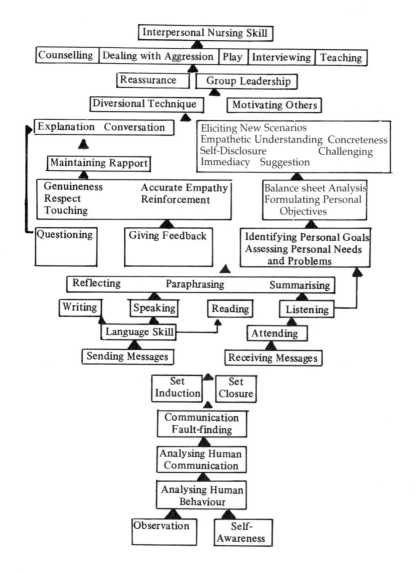

Figure 10.1 A model for organizing social skills learning.

interaction but nurses must learn them so that they can demonstrate them to the patients or carry out these activities with them. Other skills, such as reading and writing, are carried out in the absence of the author or reader respectively. Since each party in these forms of communication is separated by both distance and time, we can often forget that these are also interpersonal situations and that interaction is going on between two people. Some social skills, therefore, differ in the amount of actual face-to-face contact. Most skills described in this book are, however, characterized by face-to-face contact because this is in the very nature of nursing.

Some final comments can now be made that reflect many of the sentiments expressed in the preface. A major point expressed there is that this book would be of limited value if the reader does not bring about change in his or her own behaviour or in other people's behaviour with a view to improving the efficiency of interpersonal transactions in nursing. As a theoretical document this book can only urge the reader to attempt and practise the skills; it cannot ensure that the reader improves performance. Knowledge in itself does not bring about improved action. A book on 'riding a bicycle' will not leave the readers with an instant ability to ride a bicycle if they were unable to do so before. In the same way, a book on practical skill will not engender practical efficiency until action is taken. Once or twice in this text it has been said that skilled action is initially clumsy in the early stages of learning and that this applies equally well to social skills. This will be an obstacle to learning, requiring persistence in the face of the occasional thought that some skills are impractical. With practice, anxieties associated with initial skill learning will be alleviated and the activity will become more natural in the practice setting. In order to facilitate the learning of social skills it is useful for students of social skills and their mentors to follow some common guidelines.

FACILITATING SOCIAL SKILLS DEVELOPMENT

The development of more effective social skills for nursing practice can be achieved initially in the classroom, by simulation of human and nursing experience, but more effectively by learning in the practice learning setting. This requires that a process be adopted in which the nurse can engage in transactions with patients and colleagues and reflect on them under the guidance of a mentor (Darling, 1984). Kolb has proposed a four-stage process for learning from experience, which is relevant to both simulated and actual experience. In following this model, the facilitator promotes reflection, critical thinking, the construction of tacit knowledge and the acquisition of informed 'know-how'. Figure 10.2 shows this approach in its simplest form.

The main aim of the process is to encourage the student of social skills to think about the transaction before participation, to engage in the nursing transaction with adequate guidance and support, to think about the transaction afterwards to encourage both self-reflection and adaptation of personal strategies. This process is aided by the processes of briefing and de-briefing.

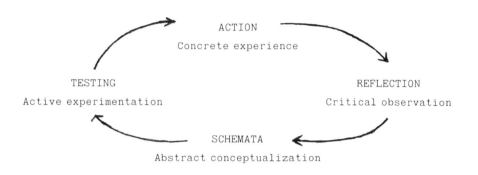

ACTION
Concrete experience

TESTING
Active experimentation

REFLECTION
Critical observation

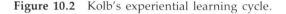

SCHEMATA
Abstract conceptualization

Figure 10.2 Kolb's experiential learning cycle.

The aims of the **briefing** session should be to:

1. Clarify the process and skills required in the nursing activity.
2. Identify any problems, constraints or restrictions the student might encounter and consider ways to alleviate them.
3. Consider the role and level of participation of the preceptor.
4. Negotiate the learning outcomes and process with the learner.

The principle of the learning contract (Mazhindu, 1990) or agreement drawn up between the student and the providers of the education is based on the assumption that the process of learning is facilitated by the willing participation of both parties and that both parties have the freedom to participate according to the personal skills and resources that are available. The learning contract is important both for the planned learning programme and the briefing session.

The **debriefing** process has been summarized by Pearson and Smith (1985) into three stages in the form of these questions:

- 'What happened?';
- 'How did the participants feel?';
- 'What does it mean?'.

A fuller description of this debriefing process and the necessary skills is not possible here and the reader is referred to an in-depth account by Pearson and Smith (1985). A second point of reference for debriefing can be equated to counselling skills. The model of counselling presented by Egan (1990) provides an interesting perspective on debriefing. This briefing/action/debriefing model is particularly useful because each stage supports another three-stage model, which emphasizes the three outcomes for social skill learning (Stammers and Patrick, 1975). They are:

1. Recognizing when the skill activities should be brought into play.
2. Being proficient at the activities and the sequencing of activities required for adequate performance.
3. Evaluating the effect/consequences of activities and making the decision when to stop the skilled action sequence.

FACILITATING INDIVIDUALIZED LEARNING PROCESSES

A final point about social skills acquisition is that it is important for the facilitator to achieve a climate that encourages ownership of the situation and empowerment in the student. The following guidelines have been suggested with particular respect to the development of student self-direction (Mast and Van Atta, 1986):

1. Build in opportunities for learners to be self-directed and responsible and to exercise their individual learning styles and preferences.
2. Encourage learners to use their current experiences as a resource for their own and other's learning.
3. Select learning material that will be applied to life tasks.
4. Create a problem-centred rather than a subject-centred orientation to learning.

Finally, I would like to encourage the reader to demonstrate unashamedly social skill when it is acquired and to teach it wherever it is necessary and required by others. Please give social skill sufficient acknowledgement by recognizing its importance and promoting its use in a sensitive and caring manner.

Nursing as a profession is characterized by continuous, persistent and intimate personal relationships. If we are to acknowledge and respect the worth of the individual human being and provide appropriate and sensible care we must learn how to relate to patients in a most proficient and helpful manner. I am tempted at this point to say, 'Good luck' but as I do not believe and cannot condone any idea that social skill learning should be haphazard or susceptible to chance, I am bound to say 'Best wishes and enjoy your practice'.

REFERENCES

Abercrombie, D. (1968) Paralanguage. *British Journal of Disorders of Communication*, **3**, 55–59. [Reprinted in *Communication in Face-to-face Interaction*, (eds J. Laver and S. Hutcheson), Penguin, Harmondsworth.

Adams, G. (1992) *Games Hong Kong People Play: A Social Psychology of the Chinese People*, TAAHK, Hong Kong.

Adderly, K. and others (1975) *Project Methods in Higher Education*, Society for Research into Higher Education, Guildford.

Anderson, E.R. (1973) *The Role of the Nurse*, Royal College of Nursing, London.

Anderson, F. (1976) *Practical Management of the Elderly*, Blackwell Scientific Publications, Oxford.

Argyle, M. (1969) *Social Interaction*, Methuen, London.

Argyle, M. (1972) *The Psychology of Interpersonal Behaviour*, 2nd edn, Penguin, Harmondsworth.

Argyle, M. (1973) *Social Encounters*, Penguin, Harmondsworth.

Argyle, M. and Dean, J. (1965) Eye contact, distance and affiliation, *Sociometry*, **28**, 173–87. [Reprinted in Argyle 1973.]

Ashworth, P. (1980) *Care to Communicate*, Royal College of Nursing, London.

Bailey, R. and Clarke, M. (1989) *Stress and Coping in Nursing*, Chapman & Hall, London.

Baker, S.J. (1955) The theory of silence, *Journal of General Psychology*, **53**, 145–67.

Bales, R.F. (1950) *Interaction Process Analysis: a Method for the Study of Small Groups*, Addison Wesley, Reading, Massachusetts.

Barnes, E. (1961) *People in Hospital*, Macmillan, London.

Baron, R.A. (1989) *Psychology*, 2nd edn, Allyn & Bacon, Boston.

Baron, R.A. (1992) *Psychology*, 3rd edn, Allyn & Bacon, Boston.

Bartlett, F.C. (1932) *Remembering: A Study of Experimental and Social Psychology*, Cambridge University Press, Cambridge.

Bateson, G. (1972) *Steps to an Ecology of Mind*, Ballantine Books, New York.

Baumeister R.F. and Tice D.M. (1986) Four selves,two motives and a substitute process self-regulation model, in *Public Self and Private Self*, (ed R.F. Baumeister), Springer-Verlag, New York.

Bavelas, A. (1950) Communication patterns in task-oriented groups. *Journal of the American Acoustical Society of America*, **22**, 725–30.

Bavelas, A., Hastorf, A.H., Gross, A.E. and Kite, W.R. (1965) Experiments on the alteration of group structure, *Journal of Experimental and Social Psychology*, **1**, 55–70.

Benner, P (1984) *From Novice to Expert: Excellence and Power in Clinical Nursing Practice*, Addison Wesley, California.

Bennis, W.G. (1976) New patterns of leadership for tomorrow's organizations, in *Management for Nurses: A Multi-disciplinary Approach*, (eds S. Stone, M.S. Berger, D. Elhart *et al.*) C.V. Mosby, St Louis.

Berman, C.M. (1977) Significance of animal play. *Nursing Mirror*, 29 December.

Berne, E. (1964) *Games People Play*, Grove Press, New York.

Berne, E. (1972) *What Do You Say After You Say Hello?*, Corgi, London.

Bernstein, B. (1959) A public language: some sociological implications of linguistic form, *British Journal of Sociology*, **10**, 311–26.

Bernstein, B. (1971) Social class, language and socialization, in *Current Trends in Linguistics*, (eds A.S. Abramson *et al.*) Mouton Press, The Hague. [Also in Brown, ·H. and Stevens, R. (1975) *Social Behaviour and Experience: Multiple Perspectives* , Hodder and Stoughton,London, in association with Open University Press.]

Berryman, J.C (1991) *Developmental Psychology and You*, British Psychological Society and Routledge, London.

Berscheid, E. and Walster, E. H. (1969) *Interpersonal Attraction*, Addison Wesley, Reading, Massachusetts.

Birch, J.A. (1978) Anxiety in nurse education. PhD Thesis, University of Newcastle.

Birchenall, P.D. (1983) Teaching interpersonal and helping skills to trainee nurse teachers: exploring the effectiveness of a course of study. MA Thesis, University of York.

Bloom, B.S. (ed.) (1956) *Taxonomy of Educational Objectives: The Classification of Educational Goals. Handbook 1: Cognitive Domain*, Mckay, New York.

Boden, M. (1977) *Artificial Intelligence and Natural Man*, Harvester Press, Hassocks.

Boore, J.R.P. (1978) *Prescription for Recovery*, Royal College of Nursing Research Series, Churchill Livingstone, Edinburgh.

Borsig, A. and Steinacker, I. (1982) Communication with the patient in the intensive care unit, *Nursing Times*, **78**(12) suppl., 1–11.

Bower, L. (1977) *The Process of Planning Nursing Care: A Model for Practice*, C.V. Mosby, St Louis.

Brammer, L. (1973) *The Helping Relationship: Process and Skills*, Prentice-Hall, Englewood Cliffs, New Jersey.

Brandes,D. and Phillips, H. (1979) *Gamesters Handbook: 140 Games for Teachers and Group Leaders*, Hutchinson, London.

Bridge, W. and Macleod Clark, J. (1981) *Communication in Nursing Care*, HM & M Publishers, Aylesbury.

Broadbent, D.E. (1985) *Perception and Communication*, Pergamon, London.

Brown, A (1986) *Group Work*, Gower Press, Aldershot.

Brown, G.W. and Rutter, M.L. (1978) The measurement of family activities and relationships: a methodological study, in *Basic Readings in Medical Sociology*, (eds D.Tuckett and J.M. Kaufert), Tavistock Publications, London.

Brown, H. and Murphy, J. (1976) *Persuasion and Coercion*, Open University Press, Milton Keynes.

Brown, R. (1976) *A First Language*, Penguin, Harmondsworth, pp. 98–115. [Also in Lee V. (ed.) (1979) *Language Development*, Croom Helm, London.]

Bruner, J. (1974) From communication to language – a psychological perspective. *Cognition*, **3**, 25–27. [Also in Lee, V. (ed.) (1979) *Language Development*, Croom Helm, London.]

Burnard, P. (1992) *Effective Communication Skills for Health Professionals*, Chapman & Hall, London.

Burton, G. (1965) *Nurse and Patient:The Influence of Human Relationships*, Tavistock Publications, London, p. 165.

Campbell, R.A. (1989) *Psychiatric Dictionary*, 6th edn, Oxford University Press, Oxford.

Cannon, W.B. (1932) *The Wisdom of the Body*, Norton, New York.

Carkhuff, R.R. (1969) *Helping and Human Relations: a Primer for Lay Helpers, Vol. 2, Practice and Research* : Holt, Rinehart and Winston, New York.

Carter, L.F. (1953) Leadership and small group behaviour, in Sherif, M. and Wilson, M.O. (eds) *Group Relations at the Crossroads*, Harpers, New York.

Cartwright, A. (1964) *Human Relations and Hospital Care*, Routledge and Kegan Paul, London.

Cattell,R.B., Eber, H.W. and Tatsuoka, M.M. (1970) *Handbook for the Sixteen Personality Factor Questionnaire*, Champaign, Institute for Personality and Ability Testing, Illinois.

Chapin, H.D. (1915) A plea for accurate statistics in childrens institutions, *Transactions of the American Pediatric Society*, **27**, 180.

Chetwyn,T (1975) How to interpret your own dreams (in one minute or less). Dell, New York.

Clinebell, H.J. (1966) *Basic Types of Pastoral Counselling*, Abingdon Press, New York.

Clift, J.D. and Clift, W.B. (1987) *Symbols of Transformations in Dreams*, Crossroad, New York.

Coghill, N.F. (1971) The West Middlesex Hospital report, in *Changing Hospitals*, (eds Wieland, G. and Leigh, H.) Tavistock, London, pp. 183–210.

Cook, M. (1970) Experiments on orientation and proxemics, *Human Relations*, **23**, 61–76.

Coxhead, D and Hiller,S (1976) *Dreams: Visions of the Night*, Avon Books, New York.

Crute, V.C., Hargie, O.D.W. and Ellis, R.A.F. (1989) An evaluation of a communication skills course for health visitor students. *Journal of Advanced Nursing*, **14**, 54.

Crystal, D. (1969) *Prosodic Systems and Intonation in English*, Cambridge University Press, Cambridge.

Dainow, S. and Bailey, C. (1988) *Developing Skills with People: Training for Person-to-Person Client Contact*, Wiley, Chichester.

Darling, L.A.W. (1984) What Do Nurses Want in a Mentor? *Journal of Nursing Administration*, October, 42–44.

Davis, J.H. (1969) *Group Performance*, Addison Wesley, London.

Department of Health and Social Security (DHSS) (1976) *The Management of Violent or Potentially Violent Hospital Patients*, HC(76), HMSO, London.

Dickson, D.A., Hargie, O. and Morrow, N.C. (1989) *Communication Skills for Health Professionals*, Chapman & Hall, London.

Douglass, L.M (1992) *The Effective Nurse: Leader and Manager*, Mosby, St Louis.

Duverger, M. (1972) *The Study of Politics*, (trans. R. Wagoner), Thomas Nelson & Sons, London.

Egan, G. (1975) *The Skilled Helper: A Model for Systematic Helping and Interpersonal Relating*, Brooks/Cole, California.

Egan, G. (1990) *The Skilled Helper: A Systematic Approach to Effective Helping*, Brooks/Cole, California.

Ehrmann, M. (1983) *Desiderata*, Souvenir Press, London.

Ellis, D.A., Hopkin, J.M., Leitch, A.G. and Crofton, J. (1979) 'Doctors orders': a controlled trail of supplementary, written information for patients. *British Medical Journal*, **1**, 456.

Elms, R.R. and Leonard, R.C. (1966) Effects of nursing approaches during admission, *Nursing Research*, **15**, 39–48.

Emerson, J. (1970) Behaviour in private places: sustaining definitions of reality in gynaecological examinations, in *Recent Sociology*, No.2, (ed. H.P. Dreitzel), Macmillan, New York, pp. 74–97.

ENB (1987) *Managing Change in Nursing Education*, English National Board for Nursing, Midwifery and Health Visiting, London.

Enelow, A.J. and Swisher, S.N. (eds) (1979) *Interviewing and Patient Care*, 2nd edn, Oxford University Press, New York.

Estabrookes, C.A and Morse, J.M (1992) Towards a theory of touch: the touching process and acquiring touching style. *Journal of Advanced Nursing*, **17**, 448–456.

Exline, R.V. and Winters, L.C. (1965) Affective relations and mutual gaze in dyads, in *Affect, Cognition and Personality*, (eds S. Tomkins and C. Izzard) Springer, New York.

Eysenck, H.J. and Eysenck S.B.J. (1975) *EPQ (Adult)*, Hodder and Stoughton, Sevenoaks.

Falbo, T. and Peplau, L.A. (1980) Power strategies in intimate relationships, *Journal of Personality and Social Psychology*, **38**, 618–28.

Faulkner, A. (1985) *Nursing: A Creative Approach.*, Baillière Tindall, London.

Faulkner, A. (1985) The organizational context of interpersonal skills in nursing, in *Interpersonal Skills in Nursing Research and Applications*, (ed. C. Kagan), Croom Helm, London.

Festinger, L. (1957) *A Theory of Cogitive Dissonance*, Row, Peterson and Co. and Stanford University Press, Stanford, California.

Fiedler, F. (1974) *Leadership and Effective Management*, Scott, Foresman and Co., Glenview, Illinois.

Flesch, R. (1964) *How to Write, Speak and Think More Effectively*, Signet Books, New York.

Francis, G.M. and Munjas, B. (1968) *Promoting Psychological Comfort*, Foundations of Nursing Series, Wm C. Brown Co.,Dubuque, Iowa.

Frank, L.K. (1957) Tactile communication, *Genetic Psychology Monographs*, **56**, 211–55.

French, H.P. (1989) Reassurance: a nursing skill?, *Journal of Advanced Nursing*, **4**, 62–64.

French, H.P. (1989) Educating the nurse practitioner: An assessment of the pre-registration preparation of nurses as an educational experience. PhD Thesis, University of Durham.

Freud, S. (1914) Further recommendations in the technique of psychoanalysis: recollection, repetition and working through, in *Collected Papers 2*, (1933), Hogarth Press, London.

Freud, S. (1940) An outline of psychoanalysis, in Strachey, J. (ed.) (1964) *Standard Edition*, **23**, 139–207.

Freud, S. (1901) in Strachey, J. (1960) The psychopathology of everyday life. *Standard Edition*, **6**.

Freud, S. (1940) in Strachey, J. (1964) An outline of psychoanalysis. *Standard Edition*, **23**.

Friedman, N. and Hoffman, S.P. (1967) Kinetic behaviour in altered clinical states: approach to objective analysis of motor behaviour during clinical interviews, *Perceptual and Motor Skill*, **24**, 52–9.

Frost, M. (1974) *Nursing Care of the Schizophrenic Patient*, Henry Kimpton, London.

Gagnon, A.J. (1983) Transcultural nursing: including it in the curriculum. *Nursing and Health Care*, **4**(3), 127–31.

Gaskell, G. and Sealy, P. (1976) *Social Psychology Block 13: Groups*, Open University Press, Milton Keynes.

Gelatt, H.B. (1962) Decision-making: A Conceptual Frame of Reference for Counselling, *Journal of Counselling Psychology*, **9**(3), 240–5.

George, J.B. (ed.) (1990) *Nursing Theories: The Base for Professional Nursing Practice*, 3rd edn, Appleton & Lange, Norwalk.

Gergen, K.J. (1969) *The Psychology of Behavior Exchange*, Addison Wesley, Reading, Massachusetts.

Gibb, C.A. (1949) The emergence of leadership in small temporary groups of men. Doctoral dissertation, University of Illinois. [Also in McKeachie, W.J. and Doyle, C.L. (1970) *Psychology*, 2nd edn, Addison Wesley, Reading, Massachusetts.]

Gibb, C.A.(1969) Leadership, in *Handbook of Social Psychology*, 4, (eds G. Lindsey and E. Aronson), Addison-Wesley, Cambridge, Massachusetts, pp. 205–81.

Gillies, D.E. (1989) *Nursing Management: A Systems Approach*, 2nd edn, W.B. Saunders, Philadelphia.

Goldman. J. J (1992) *Review of General Psychiatry*, Prentice Hall, London.

Gordon, M. (1987) *Nursing Diagnosis: Process and Application*, 2nd edn, McGraw-Hill, New York.

Gregg, D. (1955) Reassurance. *American Journal of Nursing*, **55**(2), 171–4.

Grohar-Murray, M.N. and DiGroce, H.R. (1992) *Leadership and Management in Nursing*, Appleton Lange, Connecticut.

Hall, E.T. (1959) *The Silent Language*, Doubleday, New York.

Halpin, A.W. (1965) Escape from leadership, *Journal of Education*, **11**.

Halpin, A.W. and Croft, D.B. (1963) *The Organizational Climate of Schools*, Midwest Administration Center, University of Chicago, Chicago, Illinois.

Halpin, A.W. and Winer, B.J. (1957) A factorial study of leader behaviour descriptions, in *Leader Behaviour: Its Description and Measurement*, (eds B.M. Stogdill and A.E. Coons), Research Monograph, Ohio State University, Columbus, Ohio.

Hargie, O., Saunders, C. and Dickson, D. (1981) *Social Skills in Interpersonal Communication* Croom Helm, London.

Hargie, O., Saunders, C. and Dickson, D. (1987) *Social Skills in Interpersonal Communication*, 2nd edn, Chapman & Hall, London.

Harlow, H.F. (1950) Learning and satiation of response in intrinsically motivated complex puzzle performance by monkeys. *Journal of Comparative and Physiological Psychology*, **43**, 289–94.

Harlow, H.F. (1959) Love in infant monkeys, in *Scientific American* (1974) *Papers on Socialisation and Attitudes*, W.H. Freeman, San Franciso.

Harlow, H.F. (1971) *Learning to Love*, Albion, San Francisco.

Harvey, S. and Hales-Tooke, A. (1972) *Play in Hospital*, Faber & Faber, London.

Harris, T.A. (1973) *I'm OK – You're OK*, Pan Books, London.

Hastorf, A.H. (1965) The "reinforcement' of individual actions in a group situation, in *Research in Behaviour Modification: New Developments and Implications*, (eds L. Krasner and L.P. Ullmann), Holt, Rinehart & Winston, New York.

Hayes, J. (1991) *Interpersonal Skills. Goal-directed Behaviour at Work*, Harper Collins, London.

Hays, J.S. and Larson, K.H. (1963) *Interacting with Patients*, Macmillan, New York.

Hayter, J. (1981) Territoriality as a universal need, *Journal of Advanced Nursing*, **6**, 79–85.

Hayward, J. (1975) *Information – A Prescription Against Pain*. The study of Nursing Care Project Reports, Series 2, No. 5, Royal College of Nursing, London.

Helfer, R.E. (1970) An objective comparison of the paediatric interviewing skills of freshmen and senior medical students, *Paediatrics*, **45**, 623–7.

Henderson, V. (1966) *The Nature of Nursing*, Macmillan, New York.

Hind, D. (1989) *Transferable Personal Skills; A Tutor's Manual*, Business Education Publishers, Newcastle-Upon-Tyne.

Hinsie, L.E. and Campbell, R.J. (1970) *Psychiatric Dictionary*, 4th edn, Oxford Medical Publications, Oxford.

Hockett, C.F. (1960) The origin of speech, *Scientific American*, **203**, 89–96.

Hockett, C.F. (1963) The problem of universals in language, in *Universals of Language*, (ed. J.H. Greenberg) MIT Press, Cambridge, Massachusetts.

Hockett, C.F. and Altman, S.A. (1968) A note on design features, in *Animal Communication*, Indiana University Press, Bloomington.

Hollander, E.P. and Webb, W.B. (1955) Leadership, fellowship, and friendship; an analysis of peer nominations, *Journal of Abnormal and Social Psychology*, **50**, 163–7.

Hopson, B. (1981) Counselling and helping, in *Psychology and Medicine*, (ed. Griffiths, D.) MacMillan, London.

Hull, C.L. (1943) *Principles of Behaviour*, Appleton-Century-Crofts, New York.

Hunt, J.McV. (1960) Experience and the development of motivations: some reinterpretations, *Child Development*, **31**, 489–504.

Hunt, J.M. and Marks-Maran, D.J. (1980) *Nursing Care Plans: The Nursing Process at Work*, HM & M Publishers, Aylesbury.

Hurst, K. (1985) Traditional Verses Progressive Nurse Education: A Review of the Literature, *Nurse Education Today*, **5**, 3–6.

Inskipp, F., Johns, H. and Heaviside, P. (1978) *Principles of Counselling*. A series of eight half-hour programmes for people who wish to improve their interpersonal and counselling skills. Background notes. BBC Further Education Publication, London.

Isaacs, S. (1930) *Intellectual Growth in Young Children*, Routledge & Kegan Paul, London.

Isaacs, S. (1933) *Social Development in Young Children*, Routledge & Kegan Paul, London.

Isaacs, S. (1968) *The Nursery Years*, Routledge & Kegan Paul, London.

Ivey, A.E. and Authier, R.J. (1978) *Microcounselling: Innovations in Interviewing, Counselling, Psychotherapy and Psychoeducation*, Charles C. Thomas, Springfield, Illinois.

Jack, L.M. (1934) An experimental study of ascendant behaviour in preschool children, *University of Iowa Studies in Child Welfare*, **9**, 3.

James, L.M. (1975) *Psychology for Nurses*. Study Guide for series of audiotapes, Graves Medical Audiovisual Library, Chelmsford, Essex.

Janis, I. (1958) *Psychological Stress*, John Wiley & Sons, New York.

Jennings, H.H. (1950) *Leadership and Isolation*, 2nd edn, Longmans Green, New York.

Jones, C.J. (1977) The nursing process – individualized care, *Nursing Times*, 13 October.

Jones, E.E. and Gerard, H.B. (1967) *Foundations of Social Psychology*, Wiley, New York.

Jones, S.E and Yarborough A.E. (1985) A naturalistic study of the meaning of touch, *Communication Monographs*, **52**, 19–56.

Jourard, S.M. (1966) An exploration study of body accessibility, *British Journal of Social and Clinical Psychology*, **5**, 221–31.

Kahn, J.H. (1971) *Human Growth and the Development of Personality*, 2nd edn, Pergamon Press, Oxford.

Kalish, R.A. (1966) *The Psychology of Human Behaviour*, Wadsworth Publishing, Belmont, California.

Karthwohl, D.R., *et al.* (1964) *Taxonomy of Educational Objectives: The Classification of Educational Goals. Handbook 2 Affective Domain*, Mckay, New York.

Kaul, T.J. and Parker, C.A. (1971) Suggestibility and expectancy in a counselling analogue, *Journal of Counselling Psychology*, **18**, 536–41.

Kelly, G.A. (1955) *The Psychology of Personal Constructs*, Norton, New York.

Kelman, H.C. (1967) Three processes of social influence, in *Current Perspectives in Social Psychology*, (eds E.P. Hollander, and R.G.Hunt), Oxford University Press, New York, pp. 438–46.

Keltner, N.L., Schwecke, L.H. and Bostram, C.E. (1991) *Psychiatric Nursing: A Psychotherapeutic Approach*, Mosby, St Louis.

Kendon, A. (1967) Some functions of gaze direction in social interaction, *Acta Psychologica*, **26**, 1–47.

King, I.M. (1981) *A Theory of Nursing: Systems, Concepts, Process,* John Wiley, Chichester.

Knight, M. and Field, D. (1981) Silent conspiracy: coping with dying cancer patients on acute surgical wards, *Journal of Advanced Nursing*, **6**(3), 221–9.

Kolb, D. (1976) *The Learning Style Inventory: A Technical Manual*, McBer, Boston, Massachusetts.

Kozielecki, J. (1981) *Psychological Decision Theory*, D. Reidel Publishing, Dordrecht.

Kratz, C.J. (ed.) (1979) *The Nursing Process*, Baillière Tindall, London.

Kretch, D., Crutchfield, R.S. and Ballechey, E.L. (1962) *Individual in Society*, McGraw-Hill, New York.

Kron, T. (1972) *Communication in Nursing*, 2nd edn, W.B. Saunders, Philadelphia.

Lazarus, R.S. (1966) *Psychological Stress and the Coping Process*, McGraw-Hill, London.

Leavitt, H.J. (1951) Some effects of certain patterns on group performance, *Journal of Abnormal and Social Psychology*, **46**, 38–50.

LeBon, G. (1895) *Psychologie des Foules*, F. Olean, Paris. [Translation in 1896 as *The Crowd* (trans. T. Fisher), Unwin, London.]

Lee, F.A. and Sclare, A.B. (1971) *The Modern Practical Nursing Series: Psychiatry*, Heinemann Medical, London.

Lee, V. (1976) *Social Relationships*, Open University Press, Milton Keynes.

Leininger, M. (1974) The leadership crisis in nursing: a critical problem and challenge, *Journal of Nursing Administration*, **4**(2), 2–4.

Leininger, M. (1978) *Transcultural Nursing: Concepts, Theories and Practices,*John Wiley & Sons, New York.

Leininger, M. (1989) Transcultural Nurse Specialists and Generalists: New Practitioners in Nursing, *Journal of Transcultural Nursing*, **1**(1), 6.

Lewin, K. (1947) Group decisions and social change, in *Readings in Social Psychology*, (eds T. Newcombe and E. Harley), Holt, New York.

Lewis, G.D. (1973) *Nurse-Patient Communication*, 2nd edn, Wm C. Brown, Dubuque, Iowa.

Ley, P. (1979) Memory for medical information, *British Journal of Social and Clinical Psychology*, **18**, 245–55.

Ley, P. (1988) *Communicating with Patients*, Chapman & Hall, London.

Longhorn, E.L. (1975) *Psychiatric Care and Conditions*, HM & M Publishers, Aylesbury.

Luft, J. (1969) *On Human Interaction*, National Press, Palo Alto, California.

Lyons, J. (1972) Human language, in *Non-verbal Communication*, (ed. R. Hinde) Cambridge University Press, Cambridge.

McClelland, D.C. (1975) *Power: The Inner Experience*, Irvington, New York.

McCorkle, R. (1974) Effects of touch on seriously ill patients, *Nursing Research*, **23**(2), 125–32.

McFarlane, J. and Castledine, G. (1982) *A Guide to the Practice of Nursing using the Nursing Process*, Mosby, London.

McKeachie, W.J. and Doyle, C.L. (1970) *Psychology*, 2nd edn, Addison Wesley, Reading, Massachusetts.

McNaught, A.B. and Callander, R. (1971) *Nurses Illustrated Physiology*, 2nd edn, Churchill Livingstone, Edinburgh.

McPartland, T.S. (1965) *Manual for the 'Twenty Statements' Problem*, Greater Kansas City Mental Health Foundation, Kansas City.

Mackie, L. (1979) Revitalising the nursing care plan, *Nursing Times*, **75**(34), 1440–3.

Macleod-Clark, J. (1983) Nurse–patient communication: an analysis of conversations from surgical wards, in *Nursing Research, Ten Studies in Patient Care*, (ed. J. Wilson-Barnett), John Wiley, Chichester.

Mager, R.F. (1962) *Preparing Instructional Objectives*, Fearon, Palo Alto, California.

Mann, R.D. (1959) A review of the relationships between personality and performance in small groups, *Psychological Bulletin*, **56**, 241–7.

Maslow, A. (1954) *Motivation and personality*, Harper, New York.

Mason, A. and Pratt, J. (1980) Touch. *Nursing Times*, 999–1001.

Mast, M.E. and Van Atta, M.J. (1986) Applying Adult Principles in Instructional Module Design, *Nurse Educator*, **11**(1), 35–9.

Mayers, M.G. (1972) *A Systematic Approach to the Nursing Care Plan*, Appleton-Century-Crofts, New York.

Mazhindu, G.N. (1990) Contract learning reconsidered: a critical examination of implications for application in nurse education, *Journal of Advanced Nursing*, **15**, 101–9.

Melia, K. (1981) Student nurses' accounts of their work and training: a qualitative analysis. PhD Thesis, University of Edinburgh.

Menzies, I. (1960) A case study on the functioning of social systems as a defence against anxiety. A report of the nursing service in general hospital, *Human Relations*, **13**, 13–32.

Mitchell, C. (1981) New Directions in Nursing Ethics, *Massachusetts Nurse*, **50**(7).

Moloney, M.M. (1979) *Leadership in Nursing: Theory, Strategies, Action*, C.V. Mosby, St Louis.

Montague, M.F.A. (1971) *Touching: The Human Significance of the Skin*, Columbia University Press, New York.

Moreno, J.L. (1943) Sociometry and the cultural order, *Sociometry*, **6**, 299–344.

Morris, D. (1977) *Manwatching: A Field Guide to Human Behaviour*, Triad Panther, St Albans.

Munn, N.L. (1940) The effect of knowledge of the situation upon judgement of emotion from facial expression, *Journal of Abnormal and Social Psychology*, **35**, 324–8.

Murdock, B.B. Jr (1962) The serial position effect in free recall, *Journal of Experimental Psychology*, **64**, 48.

Murray, H.A. (1943) *The Thematic Apperception Test*. Harvard University Press, Harvard.

Neill, A.S. (1961) *Summerhill*, Penguin, Harmondsworth.

Neuman, B. (1982) *The Neuman systems model: application to nursing education and practice*, Appleton-Centre, Crofts, Connecticutt.

Neuman, B. (1985) *The Neuman systems model: senior nurses*, **3**(3), Sept. p. 21.

Nichols, K. and Jenkinson, J. (1991) *Leading a Support Group*, Chapman & Hall, London.

Oland, L. (1978) The need for territoriality, in *Human Needs and the Nursing Process*, (eds A. Yura and M.B. Walsh) Appleton-Century-Crofts, New York, pp. 97–140.

Oppenheim, A.N. (1966) *Questionnaire Design and Attitude Measurement*, Heinemann, London.

Palladino, C (1989) *Developing Self-Esteem: A Positive Guide for Personal Success*, Crisp Publications, California.

Parkes, K.R. (1980a) Occupational stress among student nurses – 1: A comparison of medical and surgical wards, *Nursing Times*, **76**(25), 113–16.

Parkes, K.R. (1980b) Occupational stress among student nurses – 2: A comparison of male and female wards, *Nursing Times*, **76**(26), 117–19.

Parkin, D.M (1976) Survey of success of communication between hospital staff and patients, *Public Health*, (London), **90**, 203–209.

Parry, R. (1975) *A Guide to Counselling and Basic Psychotherapy*, Churchill Livingstone, Edinburgh.

Pearson, M. and Smith, D. (1985) Debriefing in experience-based learning, in *Reflection: Turning Experience into Learning*, (eds D. Boud, R. Keogh and D. Walker), Kogan Page, London.

Pease, A. (1984) *Body Language*, Sheldon Press, London.

Perko, J.E. and Kriegh, H.Z. (1988) Psychiatric and Mental Health Nursing; A Commitment to Care and Concern, 3rd edn, Prentice Hall International, London.

Powell, J.P. (1985) Autobiographical learning, in *Reflection: Turning Experience into Learning*, (eds D. Boud, R. Keogh and D. Walker), Kogan Page, London.

Piaget, J. (1952) *The Childs Conception of Number*, Routledge & Kegan Paul, London.

Pollack, S. and Manning, P.R. (1967) An experience in teaching and doctor–patient relationship to first-year medical students, *Journal of Medical Education*, **42**, 770–4.

Pratt, J. and Mason, A. (1981) *The Caring Touch*, HM & M, Aylesbury.

Raphael, W. (1969) *Patients and Their Hospitals*, King Edward's Hospital Fund for London, London.

Reader, G.G., Pratt, L. and Mudd, M.C. (1957) What patients expect from their doctor, *Modern Hospital*, **July**.

Reed, J. (1989) All dressed up and nowhere to go: nursing assessment in care of the elderly. PhD Thesis, Newcastle Polytechnic.

Richardson, S.A., Dohrenwend, B.S. and Klein, D. (1965) *Interviewing: Its Forms and Findings*, Basic Books, New York.

Riehl, J.P. and Roy, C. (1974) *Conceptual Models for Nursing Practice*, Appleton-Century-Crofts, New York.

Roberts, T. (1971) *A Handbook for Psychiatric Nurses*, John Wright & Sons Ltd, Bristol.

Robertson, C.M. (1987) *A Very Special Form of Teaching*, Royal College of Nursing, London.

Rogers, C.R. (1951) *Client-centred Therapy*, Houghton Mifflin, Boston.

Roper, N., Logan, W.W. and Tierney, A. (1990) *The Elements of Nursing*, Churchill Livingstone, Edinburgh.

Rotam, A. and Abbatt, F.R. (1982) *Self-Assessment for Teachers of Health Workers*, World Health Organisation, Geneva.

Rycroft, C. (1968) *Anxiety and Neurosis*, Penguin, Harmondsworth.

Sacks, H., Schegloff, E. and Jefferson, G. (1974) A simplest systematics for the organization of turn-taking for conversation, *Language*, **50**, 696–735.

Sandstrom, C.I. (1966) *The Psychology of Childhood and Adolescence*, Penguin, Harmondsworth.

Sarafino, E.P (1990) *Health Psychology: Biosychosocial Interactions*, Wiley, New York.

Sarnoff, I. and Zimbardo, P.C. (1961) Anxiety, fear and social facilitation, *Journal of Abnormal and Social Psychology*, **62**, 356–63.

Scandinavian Service School (1983) *Putting Patients First*, Time Manager International, Solihull.

Schachter, S. (1959) *The Psychology of Affiliation*, Stanford University Press, Palo Alto.

Scheier, M.F., Weintraub, J.K. and Carver, C.S. (1986) Coping with Stress: Divergent strategies of optimists and pessimists, *Journal of Personality and Social Psychology*, **51**, 1257–64.

Schon, D. (1987) *Educating the Reflective Practitioner*, Jossey Bass, San Francisco.

Sherif, M. (1936) *The Psychology of Social Norms*, Harper, New York.

Sherif, M.O. and Sherif, C. (1953) *Groups in Harmony and Tension*, Harper, New York.

Sherif, M. *et al.* (1961) *Intergroup Conflict and Co-operation*, Oklahoma University Book Exchange, Oklahoma.

Siegel, L. and Siegel, L. (1965) Educational set: a determinant of acquisition, *Journal of Educational Psychology*, **56**, 1–12.

Sim, M. (1969) *Guide to Psychiatry*, 2nd edn, Churchill Livingstone, Edinburgh.

Simpson, E.J. (1966) The classification of educational objectives: psychomotor domain, in *Final Report on Vocational and Technical Education Contract OE-04*, University of Illinois College of Education, Chicago.

Simpson, J.A. and Weiner, E.S.C. (1989) *The Oxford English Dictionary*, 2nd edn, Clarendon. Oxford.

Sissons, M. (1971) *The Psychology of Social Class*, Open University Press, Milton Keynes.

Skinner, B.F. (1953) *Science and Human Behaviour*, Collier-Macmillan, London.

Snow, C. (1977) The development of conversation between mothers and babies, *Journal of Child Language*, **4**, 1–22.

Sommer, R. (1965) Further studies of small group ecology, *Sociometry*, **28**, 33–38.

South East Thames Regional Health Authority (1980) *Guidelines for the Nursing Management of Violence*, Bethlem Royal Hospital and the Maudsley Hospital, London. [Film and illustrated booklet also available from the Regional Health Authority.]

Spelman, M.S., Ley, P. and Jones, C. (1966) How do we improve doctor–patient communication in our hospitals? *World Hospitals*, **2**, 126–34.

Stammers, R. and Patrick, J. (1975) *The Psychology of Training*, Methuen, London.

Stanton, M., Paul, C. and Reeves, J.S. (1990) An overview of the nursing process, in *Nursing Theories:The Base for Professional Nursing Practice*, (ed. J.B.George), Appleton & Lange, Norwalk, Connecticut.

Steinaker, N. and Bell, M.R. (1975) A proposed taxonomy of educational objectives: the experiential domain, *Educational Technology*, **January**, 14–16.

Stevens, B. (1975) *The Nurse as Executive*, Contemporary Publishing, Wakefield, Massachusetts.

Stevens, R. (1975) *Interpersonal Communication*, Open University Press, Milton Keynes.

Stockwell, F. (1972) *The Unpopular Patient*. Royal College of Nursing Study of Nursing Care Research Project, Series 1, No.2 Royal College of Nursing, London.

Strong, S.R. (1970) Causal attribution in counselling and psychotherapy, *Journal of Counselling Psychology*, **17**, 388–99.

Sullivan, H.S. (1954) *The Psychiatric Interview*, Norton, New York.

Swider, S.M., McElmurry, B. and Yarling, R.R. (1985) Ethical decision-making in bureaucratic context by senior nursing students, *Nursing Research*, **34**(2), 108–12.

Talbot, F. (1941) Discussion, *Transactions of the American Paediatric Society*, **62**, 469.

Tannebaum, R. and Schmidt, W.H. (1958) How to choose a leadership pattern, *Harvard Business Reviews*, **36**(2), 95–101.

Taylor, C., Lillis, C. and LeMone, P. (1989) *Fundamentals of Nursing*, Lippincott, Philadelphia.

Taylor, R.B (1988) *Human Territorial Functioning*, Cambridge University Press, Cambridge.

Teasdale, K. (1989) The concept of reassurance in nursing, *Journal of Advanced Nursing*, **14**, 44–50.

Tedeschi, J.T. (1986) Private and Public Self, in Baumeister, R.F. (ed) *Public Self and Private Self*, Springer-Verlag, New York.

Thomson, B. and Bridge, W. (1982) *Teaching Patient Care*, HM & M Publishers, Aylesbury.

Thorndike, R.L. and Hagen, E.P. (1977) *Measurement and Evaluation in Psychology and Education*, 4th edn, John Wiley & Sons, New York.

Travelbee, J. (1966) *Interpersonal Aspects of Nursing*, F.A. Davis, Philadelphia.

Turney, C., Cairns, L.G., Williams, G. *et al.*(1974) *Sydney Micro Skills: Series 1 Handbook*, Sydney University Press, Sydney, Australia.

Turney, C., Owens, L.C., Hatton, N., Williams, G. *et al.*(1976) *Sydney Micro Skills: Series 2 Handbook*, Sydney University Press, Sydney, Australia.

Ulisse, G.C. (1978) *POMR: Application to Nursing Records*, Addison Wesley, Menlo Park, California.

Valentine, M. (1965) *An Introduction to Psychiatry*, Churchill Livingstone, Edinburgh.

Volicer, B.J. (1974) Patients perceptions of stressful events associated with hospitalization, *Nursing Research*, **23**(3), 235–8.

Wason, P.C. (1968) Reasoning about a rule, *Quarterly Journal of Experimental Psychology*, **20**, 273–81.

Watson, J.B. (1925) *Behaviourism*, Norton, New York.

Wattley and Muller (1987) Teaching Psychology to Nurses, in *Nurse Education: Research and Developments*, (ed. Davis, B.) Croom Helm, London.

Weiner, B. (1989) *Human Motivation*, Erlbaum, Hillsdale, New Jersey.

Weinhold, B.K. and Elliott, L.C. (1979) *Transpersonal Communication: How to Establish Contact with Yourself and Others*, Prentice-Hall, Englewood Cliffs, New Jersey.

Weller, B.F. (1980) *Helping Sick Children, Play*, Baillière-Tindall, London.

White, R. and Ewan, C. (1991) *Clinical Teaching in Nursing*, Chapman & Hall, London.

White, R.K. and Lippitt, R. (1960) *Autocracy and Democracy*, Harper, New York.

Whorf, B.L. (1952) *Collected Papers on Metalinguistics*, Department of State, Foreign Service Institute, Washington DC.

Whorf, B.L. (1956) *Language, Thought and Reality*, MIT Press, Cambridge, Massachusetts.

Wilkinson, J. and Canter, S. (1982) *Social Skills Training Manual: Assessment, Programme Design and Management of Training*, Wiley, Chichester.

Wilson-Barnett, J. (1979) *Stress in Hospital*, Churchill Livingstone, Edinburgh.

Wilson-Barnett, J. and Carrigy, A. (1978) Factors affecting patients' responses to hospitalisation, *Journal of Advanced Nursing*, **3**, 221–8.

Winefield, H.R. and Peay, M.Y. (1980) *Behavioural Science in Medicine*, Allen and Unwin (London) and Beaconsfield Publishers (Beaconsfield).

Woodworth, R.S. and Marquis, D.G. (1949) *Psychology: A Study of Mental Life*, Methuen, London.

Wooldridge, P., Skipper, J. and Leonard, R.C. (1968) *Behavioural Science, Social Practice and the Nursing Profession*, Press of Case Western Reserve, Cleveland, Ohio.

Wrightsman, L. (1960) Effects of waiting with others on changes in level of felt anxiety, *Journal of Abnormal and Social Psychology*, **61**, 216–22.

Yablonsky, L. (1962) The violent gang as a near-group, in *The Violent Gang*, Macmillan, New York.

Zajonc, R.B. and Sales, S.M. (1966) Social facilitation of dominant and subordinate responses, *Journal of Experimental Social Psychology*, **2**, 160–8.

Zander, K.S., Bower, K.A., Foster, S.D., *et al.* (eds) (1978) *Practical Manual for Patient Teaching*, C.V. Mosby, St Louis.

Zimbardo, P. and Ebbesen, E.B. (1970) *Influencing Attitudes and Changing Behaviour*, Addison Wesley, Reading, Massachusetts.

Zurcher, L.A. (1977) *The Mutable Self: A Self-concept for Social Change*, Sage Publications, California.

INDEX

Page numbers appearing in **bold** refer to figures, and page numbers appearing in *italic* refer to tables.

A Basic Introduction to Speech Perception

A Volume in

The Speech Science Series

Series Editor: Raymond D. Kent, Ph.D.